Baby Dance

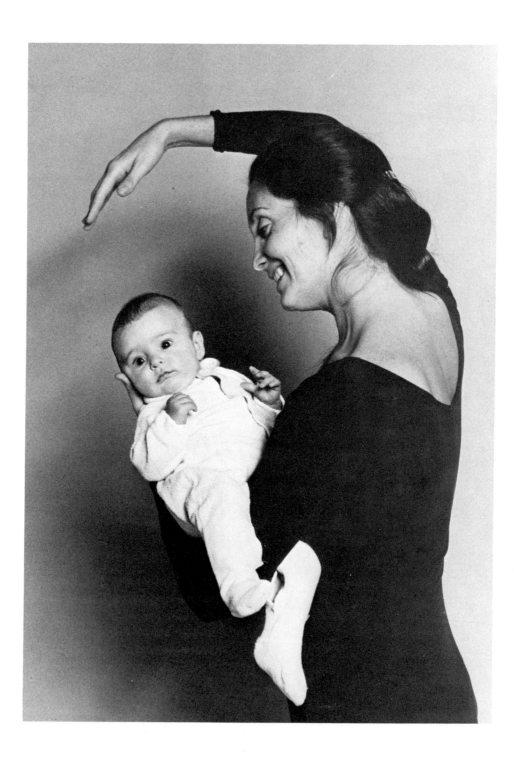

Margaret Christy
440

~~Heidi~~

Baby Dance

A comprehensive guide
to prenatal and
postpartum exercise

Elysa Markowitz
& Howard Brainen

Anatomical drawings by Len Gray

Prentice Hall Inc., Englewood Cliffs, New Jersey

Book design by Joan Ann Jacobus
Art Director: Hal Siegel

Photographs on the following pages by Ilene Segalove:
pages 66, 67, 73, 74, 76, 81, 82, 85,
90, 92, 95, 96, 98, 100, and 102.
All other photographs by Howard Brainen.

Address inquiries to Prentice-Hall, Inc.,
Englewood Cliffs, N.J. 07632
Printed in the United States of America
Prentice-Hall International, Inc., London
Prentice-Hall of Australia, Pty. Ltd., Sydney
Prentice-Hall of Canada, Ltd., Toronto
Prentice-Hall of India Private Ltd., New Delhi
Prentice-Hall of Japan, Inc., Tokyo
Prentice-Hall of Southeast Asia Pte. Ltd., Singapore
Whitehall Books Limited, Wellington, New Zealand
10 9 8 7 6 5 4 3 2 1

Library of Congress Cataloging in Publication Data
Markowitz, Elysa, date,
   Baby dance.
   Bibliography: p.
   1.   Prenatal care.   2.   Exercise for women.
3.   Pregnancy.   4.   Childbirth.   5.   Postnatal care.
6.   Infants (Newborn)—Care and hygiene.
I.   Brainen, Howard, date, joint author.
II.   Title.
RG558.7.M37   1980   618.2'4   79-24815
ISBN 0-13-055657-2

I dedicate this book to my daughter,
Anna Rachael Markowitz,
whose conception gave life to our Baby Dance.

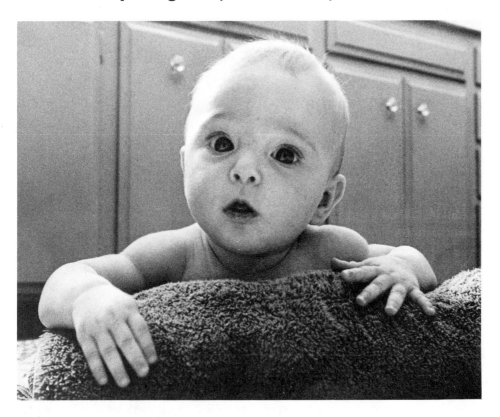

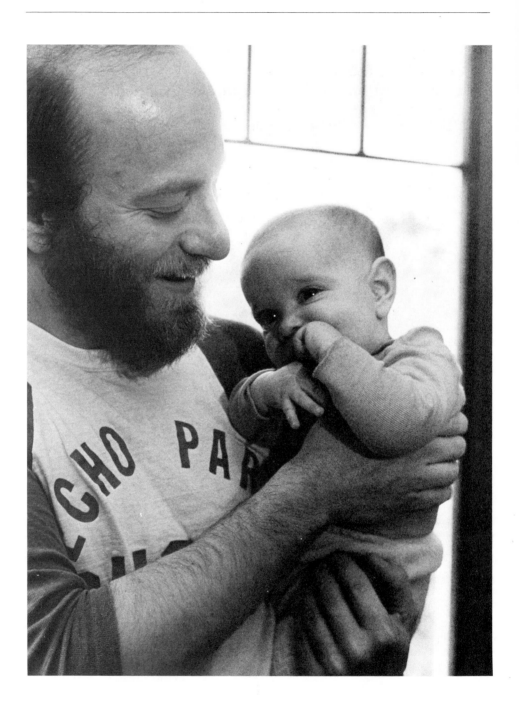

Contents

Author's acknowledgements

As I look back over the last three years, many people and incidents play back, each adding another facet to this book. I wish to acknowledge these wonderful people for their help, support, and encouragement.

A special thanks to Moe and Lucille Markowitz, my parents. They have been a blessing and a godsend, providing support for my work and being golden grandparents to Anna.

Also deserving recognition are the people who made this book possible by their presence, time, and interest, and whose faces you see in this book: Nancy Weinraub; Audrey and her son Michael Wegner; Lauren, Jules, and their daughter Mia Weinseider; Mickey Selwin; Ron, Arminda, and their son Ryan Snyder; Susan, Doug, and their daughter Tiffany Goodall; Dr. Lusk; and Dr. Boyd Cooper (for his foreword to this book).

Along the way were friends who read the manuscript and offered constructive comments, edited, or helped in the preparation of the final text. I wish to thank Ilene Segalove, Dan Goleman, Lucia Capacchione, Abbey Duncan, Margaret Ryan, Mariana Fitzpatrick, Dr. Clifton J. Strauss, Nancy Fitzgerald, Ramona Amador, Sue Yackley, Jenny Woods, and Peggy Wilvert.

To all the women and couples in my classes who have shared their pregnancy, birth, and children, a heartfelt thanks.

Last, but by far not least, one of the most significant persons involved in the making of this book is Howard Brainen, my colleague and friend, who gave his time and energy lovingly and patiently.

Elysa Markowitz

Photographer's acknowledgements

My close involvement with *Baby Dance* during the last three years has been a rich, rewarding experience. There have been many people who helped along the way, and they deserve a large vote of thanks and gratitude.

For their friendship and patience with me at the Lincoln Street house, Abbey Duncan and Bob Clary; for her radiance, Mickey Selwyn, the first midwife I ever observed in action; Jeannine Parvati and Michael Medvin for their inspiration, high energy and wisdom; Dan Bessie for his guidance; all our wonderful models, who took time out of their busy lives to be a part of *Baby Dance*—we couldn't have done it without them; at Prentice-Hall, Mariana Fitzpatrick and Hal Siegel for their enthusiasm and input.

A special word of appreciation to my lab technicians, George P. Post and Alex Cheung, whose patience and dedication helped keep me and my share of this project together.

And most of all, thanks to Elysa and Anna. Elysa *is Baby Dance*. Her ideas, her vitality, and her clarity have greatly enriched my life. Knowing Anna from the beginning—witnessing her spirit enter the world, watching her grow, communicating with her before words—has been both a nourishment and a delight.

Howard Brainen

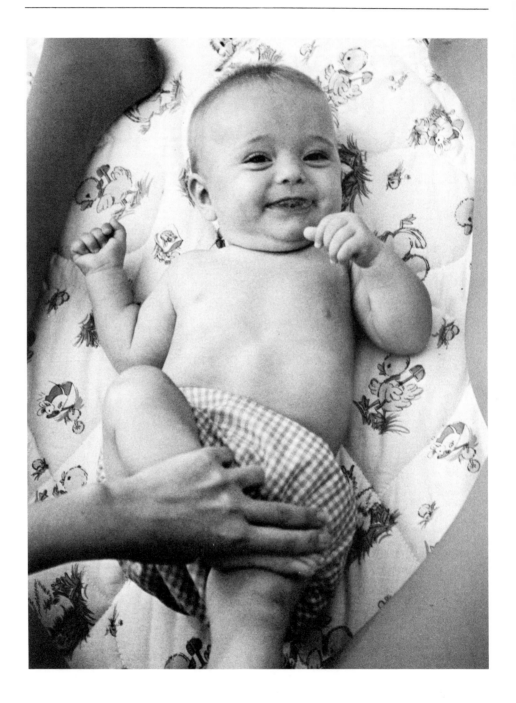

Foreword
by Boyd Cooper, M.D.

Modern obstetrics seems to have brought us full circle from primitive times, returning us to nature's way. Thanks to advanced medical knowledge, childbirth today is not only safer but simpler. We now have the capability of differentiating between high- and low-risk pregnancy. Most present-day pregnancies can be handled in a natural way, without medical interference, provided medical expertise is immediately available.

In *Baby Dance*, Ms. Markowitz emphasizes the importance of overall preparedness for birth. If modern woman is to have her baby as easily as her primitive sisters, she must be in good physical health, properly nourished, and knowledgeable about what to expect from herself and her body. The role of exercise as a way to fitness is stressed: after all, primitive woman was a much more physically active creature than her twentieth-century counterpart. The prenatal and postpartum exercises contained in this book are designed to promote a comfortable pregnancy, facilitate a natural, easy labor, and enhance a rapid recovery.

Ms. Markowitz brings both personal and professional expertise to these pages. She has worked with obstetricians and assisted with hospital and home deliveries. She has interviewed numerous pregnant women and compared their stories with the realities of her own birth experience. Her light touch and ability to share give *Baby Dance* a delightfully fresh and personal quality.

In a time when young people are endeavoring to gain self-knowledge, Ms. Markowitz has managed to get in touch with herself and life through her pregnancy. She has made having a baby a meaningful inner experience, as opposed to an externally controlled medical happening.

Introduction

This book grew out of a need I felt to combine quality information about movement and about pregnancy. My own pregnancy motivated me to find out all I could. The available books on exercise seemed incomplete. None of them mentioned the coach. Information on comfort measures during the nine months of pregnancy was sparse. There was little to read that correlated exercise and anatomy. I wanted to know how prenatal exercise related to birth preparation, how it could help during the actual labor process. I wanted to learn what to do when the baby arrived. How soon could I resume exercising? What movements would be safe for me and the baby? How could I include my newborn while getting myself back in shape?

Information was scattered and in some instances nonexistent. I decided to write a book. The process took over three years, from "conception" to "birth." As with a baby, the gestation period was well worth the wait. It helped me mature as a woman/writer/instructor.

During my pregnancy I found that one of my most important tasks was to establish priorities. Mine were as follows:

o To be calm and relaxed in order to create a healthy baby.
o To surround myself with people who were supportive of my pregnancy.
o To prepare for childbirth by learning all I could.

Focusing on my own wants helped. I was able to create support groups around me through my classes. My pregnancy was a nurturing and positive time, culminating in the successful birth of a healthy, wonderful baby girl.

I encourage all of you to set priorities. Find supportive people—your husband, friends, a sympathetic doctor—and make your "baby dance" a time of health and learning.

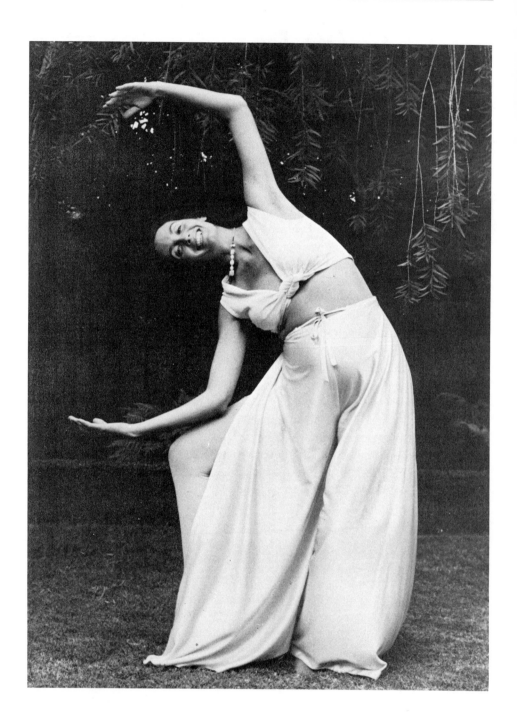

1. *Comfort tips during pregnancy*

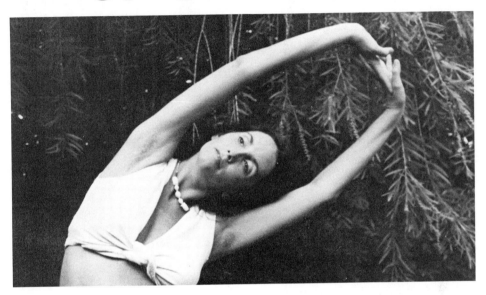

I loved being pregnant. I felt creative, alive, special, connected with a very pure part of myself. It was a time for introspection, yet I never felt really alone. My baby was always with me.

It was an active nine months. When I found out that I was pregnant, I was working with movement therapy, teaching children's dance, and performing for children's theater. I wanted to continue dancing and teaching but I didn't know if this would hurt me or the baby. I decided to find out all I could. I enrolled in childbirth classes and talked to many teachers. I questioned pregnant women and mothers I met in supermarkets. I read books. One book in particular changed my life: Jeannine Medvin's *Prenatal Yoga and Natural Birth*. Because of it, I started to exercise daily, using gentle movements. This led to teaching my own prenatal exercise class, combining yoga, tai chi, ballet, and dance movements that I found safe. This was a new kind of dancing for me: quiet, flowing—a baby dance.

By my sixth month I had finished one childbirth course and was enrolled in a program to become a certified childbirth educator. My training was completed by the time I gave birth. During those last months I took a third series of childbirth classes. You can see how much I wanted to be prepared! I also made two 16mm color films, *Prenatal Exercise* (20 minutes) and *Baby Dance* (15 minutes), which I filmed during my eighth month. They were inspired by a close friend of mine who saw me dancing when I was very pregnant.

Both of my films are now being distributed nationally and shown in doctors' offices to encourage exercise. They have helped me reach a larger group of women than my classes. They express my enthusiasm about pregnancy—as a time of joy and well-being, a well-being that is enhanced by healthful motion, good nutrition, and a positive attitude. Because of my belief in the importance of exercise in pregnancy, I created the exercise program presented in this book. I see such exercise as affecting birth and beyond, helping you move through your pregnancy, facilitating birth, and providing gentle movements to share with your newborn.

My various prenatal activities brought me in contact with many pregnant women. It was a time of openness and support. We would talk for hours about our feelings, our fears, and how we were learning and growing from the whole process. Out of these discussions came many facts about nutrition, helpful hints on how to avoid or minimize certain discomforts, and other useful information. I would like to share these with you here.

As you read this chapter, pick out the advice that works for you. Each of us has her own experience to relate to during pregnancy. You can make this a time of unease and anxiety, or a time to enjoy, a time of new, exciting experiences and events. The choice is yours.

Every pregnancy is different.

Every woman is unique.

You are not sick. You are pregnant. You are special. Enjoy!!

THE FIRST TRIMESTER

Establishing Whether You're Pregnant

The first trimester for most women is a time of dramatic change. Yet some women don't realize they are pregnant until the second or third month. Missing a period isn't always conclusive evidence. I had a suspicion I was pregnant from several signs. I was constantly tired. My breasts felt sore and tender. Before my pregnancy, I had become accustomed to checking out my cervix (the opening of the uterus) to see what changes my body was experiencing. So when my period was two weeks overdue, I felt my cervix and noticed that it felt less resilient than usual. I immediately decided to go to a women's clinic and have a pregnancy test. The results were positive. Usually a woman can determine whether or not she is pregnant by six weeks. By then there should be sufficient evidence of a hormone called human chorionic gonadotropin (HCG) in the urine. This hormone is present only during pregnancy and it is what most pregnancy tests look for.

I felt excited but at the same time nervous. Was this the right time in my life to have a baby? Did I really want to be a mother? How would a baby affect my career? I knew I was faced with a very important decision, one each woman must make for herself and one she must make wisely and maturely. Motherhood is a big step in any woman's life.

Prenatal Care

My next step was to find good prenatal care. Many communities have a family planning center. Check for other resources in your area. Obstetricians are easy to find in the phone book, but you should shop around for one who will be supportive of the kind of birth experience you want. Most of us are not going to have 8 or 10 children, so we want to make the most out of every birth we have!

I decided to use the county public health clinic. They had a special clinic for pregnant women which provided me with fine care. One of the reasons for early prenatal care is to find out if your body needs any nutritional supplements. A blood test confirmed that my iron count was low and that I was slightly anemic, which accounted for part of my fatigue. I started to take iron pills and drink a super homemade protein/iron smoothie. My recipes varied but the basic ingredients were these: some kind of fruit juice or herb tea, a banana, molasses, brewer's yeast, sesame seeds (soaked overnight or ground in a coffee grinder—a great source of calcium), cinnamon or vanilla for flavoring, and a couple of tablespoons of protein powder. In three months I brought my iron count up two points.

During every appointment at your doctor's office or clinic your urine will be examined for a number of different things: protein, sugar, ketones. Ask why. The more you know about your pregnancy the better you can take care of yourself. Your weight will also be recorded to be sure you are gaining at the proper rate for your body size. Your blood type will be checked to find out if you are RH positive or negative. If you are negative, ask your doctor what that means. Many doctors want their RH negative mothers to have a rhogam shot right after the baby is born. They'll explain the reason for this.

Early Body Changes

During the first months of pregnancy, your body will begin to transform itself. Your breasts will grow larger. The hormones estrogen and progesterone will be working overtime to prepare them for feeding the baby. You might gain over a pound in your breasts alone! I enjoyed the feeling of full, round breasts. I found I had to wear a bra, though. My breasts felt sore without proper support.

Another change you might notice is the frequency with which you have to visit the toilet. This is because your uterus is growing and beginning to press against your bladder. The uterine walls have already gotten thicker to feed the fertilized egg as it embeds into the uterine tissue. I found myself constantly heading for the bathroom, especially at night.

Your cervix will continue to change also. Because of the increased blood flow and hormones, the cervix and vagina will become softer and puffier. You might notice an increase in vaginal secretions. Make sure that you aren't experiencing any itching, burning, or unpleasant odors. They could indicate an infection and should be checked by your doctor.

Sex During Pregnancy

During the first month of pregnancy, your body will make a mucous plug to fill up the opening of the cervix. This plug helps to seal the baby off from the outside world. The baby has double protection: first, from the amniotic sac, filled with amniotic fluid, which surrounds the growing fetus like a pressurized chamber; and second, from the mucous plug keeping the cervix closed and safe from "outside invaders." Knowing this relieved my anxieties about making love while pregnant as well as my partner's when he was informed. We both knew the baby wouldn't be hurt by intercourse.

If you notice a tinge of pink after intercourse, this is no cause for alarm.

A few capillaries from your cervix or vaginal wall may have been bumped or bruised. However, if you notice any bright red or profuse bleeding, call your doctor immediately! This could be an indication of something much more serious.

Sex was very different during pregnancy. Once my belly started growing, the missionary position became uncomfortable. You might feel that way, too. Look for new positions, perhaps lying on your side or sitting up. Not all the women I have talked with enjoyed sex during their pregnancy. It's a highly individual matter. Respect your feelings, whatever they are. In my case, perhaps the "safety" of knowing I couldn't get pregnant released a lot of tension. I found sex to be wonderful. As the baby got larger, I did have some concerns that orgasm might hurt it, but the books I read said that the baby wouldn't be negatively affected by climaxing. In fact, I learned that sex would increase circulation to my pelvis and help relieve backaches.

During the last few months I wanted to make love gently. Playing romantic music added a richness to the environment, as well as a rhythm with which to make love. This is definitely a time for experimentation. I suggest that you and your partner talk about your sexual fantasies and find out what positions feel good. Try different ways of cuddling and touching each other. Elizabeth Bing and Libby Colman's *Making Love During Pregnancy* is a wonderful book to read aloud. It helps to break the ice about sex and tells what to do or expect during the different trimesters. It also might help relieve any fears you may have about your feelings.

Mood Shifts During Pregnancy

Most women feel more moody during pregnancy. If you could see what your hormones are doing, you'd know why you seem to have a roller coaster inside you. I remember how insignificant little events would bring me to tears.

These hormone changes also have their positive side. As a pregnant woman, you are more open to experiencing your feelings. It is a wonderful opportunity to see the child in you and relate to that part of yourself. You will be dealing with your own child soon enough. Respect your feelings, and take responsibility for them, too. Avoid blaming others for your mood shifts. Pregnancy is a challenging time to experience your vulnerability. We spend most of our time protecting ourselves; let this be a time to acknowledge your softness and allow others to respond to it. I found those about me were very receptive when I let them share my hurt and disappointments. Let others in on your joy and pleasures too!

Tension Headaches

Pregnant women seem especially susceptible to headaches. Perhaps it is because of hormonal changes, increased circulation in the body, or an increased sensitivity to the environment. When headaches occur, you will want to avoid taking most commercial headache remedies. As a general practice, consult with your doctor before taking medication of any kind. Many different sources advise pregnant women not to take aspirin. It may be harmful to the mother as well as the baby. In fact, most headache medicines are best left on the shelf while you are pregnant. What are the alternatives? Lying down may help. The cause could simply be fatigue. Try to relax all over. Some women find taking a bath relieves the pain. Or you might brew yourself a cup of calming herb tea. (See the charts at the end of this chapter.) Perhaps a light snack will do the trick.

I found it helpful to examine possible sources of tension. Breathing also helped me relax. I would sit down and focus on my breath going in and out. Often this would make my headache melt away. If your discomfort continues, call your doctor and ask him what is safe to take.

Changes in Circulation and How They Affect You

Did you know that a pregnant woman filters between 30 to 45 percent more blood for herself and the baby before her pregnancy is over? This means that between one-third and one-half more fluid than normal will be going through your body while you are pregnant. Does that help to explain why you feel warmer? Your whole capillary system is circulating more blood. I remember constantly taking off my sweater while everyone else was putting theirs on.

This increase in circulation also helps to explain why you are so thirsty. You need to drink more fluids while you are pregnant, to help keep your filtering systems open—especially your intestines.

Fluids are also helpful for avoiding constipation, which can be a problem during pregnancy. I remember I would go to sleep with a jug of water next to my bed. I found that eating a lot of fresh fruits and adding high fiber foods like bran or salads to my diet helped fight constipation too. I also tried to walk and exercise more. Some of the herb teas helped too. A brew of peppermint, chamomile, or sometimes comfrey was a refreshing way to start the day. My system liked the gentle warm wake-up—a wonderful substitute for caffeine drinks. Besides, I had read that caffeine inhibits the absorption of iron. I decided to encourage all the iron I ate to stay in my body to help me and the baby.

Morning Sickness

If you are experiencing nausea or vomiting, think of it as a sign that your body needs to "clean house" rather than as a sickness. Eating small amounts of food often during the day, especially fruit or foods high in protein, might help. Dry crackers or toast can be eaten in the morning before you get out of bed. Try treating yourself to a glass of sparkling cider or bubbly mineral water in a fine wine glass. It helps to treat yourself elegantly, even though you may be feeling miserable. And remember, it will all be over soon. Most women are through vomiting by their third to fifth month and start to feel terrific!

Several doctors I've talked with feel that morning sickness is the liver's way of calling for help. You might want to look up remedies for an overworked liver—for example, taking vitamin B supplements. Vitamin B-6 or B-12 is often suggested as a remedy. I enjoyed drinking fruit and vegetable juices to "feed my liver" and to put fresh minerals and vitamins into my body quickly. (I would dilute the juices with water so that they weren't as sweet.) My system found citrus juice too harsh, but experiment for yourself; some systems can handle undiluted orange or grapefruit juice.

The Two No-No's: Cigarettes and Alcohol

One vivid memory I have from my third month on is that cigarette smoke made me nauseated. One whiff was enough to make me turn green.

For those of you who smoke, this is a perfect time to stop. If you have ever had the desire to quit, you now have the strongest possible motive. Many women who came to my classes stopped smoking while they were pregnant. It was a gift they gave to their babies. Several studies have shown that women who smoke have smaller babies. Smaller infants tend to have fewer defenses. What's more, every time you inhale, you deprive your baby of oxygen, since the nicotine constricts your blood vessels. I used to smoke and, believe me, I know how hard it is to quit. But, I had promised myself I would quit *before* I got pregnant and, once I made up my mind that I was going to stop, I did. I found combining herbs like lavender, coltsfoot, mullein, yerba buena, and red raspberry into "tobacco" which I rolled up in paper helped. It gave me something to puff on while I was going through the nicotine withdrawal. I still thank myself for quitting, for offering myself a gift of time and money while giving my child the gift of health.

There has been a lot of current publicity about pregnant women and alcohol. The FDA is considering putting labels on beer, wine, and hard liquor warning that alcohol is dangerous for pregnant women. Try toasting your unborn baby with sparkling cider or bubbly mineral water instead.

Bleeding Gums

Some women experience bleeding gums during pregnancy. I found that whenever I brushed my teeth I would start to bleed. I was relieved to learn that all the mucous membranes tend to be more sensitive during pregnancy. A friend of mine suggested that I eat citrus fruits, red and green peppers, and other foods high in vitamin C. The bleeding stopped within a week. I was very grateful for that simple, yet effective advice.

THE MIDDLE TRIMESTER

Changes in Your Internal Organs

What happens to your organs as the baby grows? How will they have enough room? I found myself asking such questions when I was pregnant. The first childbirth preparation class I attended was in my fifth month. I'm glad I went that early. The teacher showed us some charts which gave me some answers. Below are two drawings of a woman's anatomy, one before and one during pregnancy, which clarify what is happening inside you.

In these drawings you can see the difference between a nonpregnant woman and one who is five months pregnant. In Figure 1–1, all the organs have plenty of space. The uterus, intestines, stomach, and lungs each have their own private "rooms." The same is true for the bladder. Now look at the change in Figure 1–2. The baby has grown and is above the bladder, applying pressure from the top. The 26 feet or so of the intestines are definitely being squeezed. At five months there is also less space for the stomach and lungs. Note the fine "cradle" a

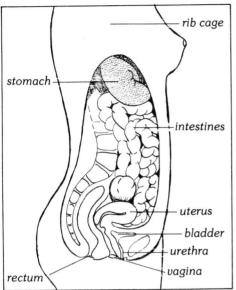

Figure 1-1. *Nonpregnant anatomy*

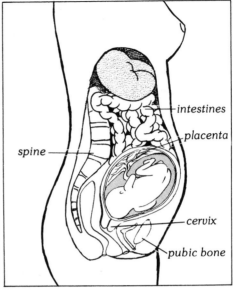

Figure 1-2. *Five months pregnant*

woman's body builds. It is amazing to observe the changes nature makes in us to support and nourish the growth of new life! Note also that the pregnant woman gains weight in her thighs and buttocks to support the extra weight from the baby's development.

Importance of Nutrition

A look at Figures 1–1 and 1–2 helps explain why constipation or gas can be a problem during pregnancy. There just isn't as much space in those 26 or so feet of tubing for your food to pass through. One area in your diet to check is how you are combining your foods. It's not only what you eat, it's what you eat *together* that produces gas. Beans and fried or greasy foods are prime offenders. Your body will tell you in no uncertain terms what it will and will *not* tolerate. You'll feel much better when you have identified the foods, or combinations of foods, that are causing you discomfort.

Relieving gas pains can be tricky. You might try the knee-chest position (called here *The Turtle*; see Chapter 2). It usually works quickly and efficiently. *Pelvic Rocks* (see Chapter 2) also move gas and food through the intestines.

Charcoal tablets were recommended by a friend of mine who had used them with great success to relieve gas during two pregnancies. You can buy them at the drugstore.

During my pregnancy my diet was better than it had been in years. This was because I checked to see what was in the foods I was eating. After all, I wanted to build a healthy baby. At the same time, I was nurturing myself. Take advantage of your pregnancy to establish better eating habits while giving your baby the best start you can inside you! The following nutrient chart will help.

WHAT YOUR BABY NEEDS TO GROW

Nutrient and Effects on Baby

Protein
Placental growth, helps to build new tissues in vagina, uterus, and blood. Contains all essential amino acids.

Iron
Probably the most important mineral for the pregnant woman. One-third of the iron is absorbed by and used to form the baby's blood.

Folic Acid
Aids in iron use, blood volume.

Calcium
Needed for the formation of good bones and teeth in the baby.

Folacin
Necessary for proper cell division and growth of organism.

Food Sources

See Protein Chart

Organ meats, meats, fish, poultry, blackstrap molasses, cherry juice, watermelon, green leafy vegetables, raw spinach (in salads), dried fruits, raisins, dessicated liver.

800 micrograms per day. Dark leafy greens, organ meats, brewer's yeast, root vegetables, whole grains, oysters, salmon, whole milk, dates, raw elderberries.

Whole milk, milk products, dark leafy greens, shellfish, salmon, molasses, prunes, dried apricots, raisins, cooked rhubarb, sesame seeds, oranges, watermelon, papayas, bone meal and dolomite, carrots.

Orange juice, garbanzo beans, kidney beans, soybeans, spinach, romaine lettuce, cabbage, sweet potatoes.

*Nutrient and Effects on Baby*___   ## *Food Sources*___

Vitamin A
Helps fight infection in the eyes, controls tooth enamel formation as well as eye growth. Aids functioning of the cells of the skin and mucous membranes.

Dried apricots, cantaloupe, cherries, raw elderberries, pink grapefruit, nectarines, papayas, peaches, stewed prunes, liver, eggs, yellow vegetables, green vegetables, whole milk and milk products, fish liver oil.

Vitamin B Complex
Helps control nausea of early pregnancy. Deficiency can contribute to toxemia. Anti-stress vitamin.

Brewer's yeast, whole grains, legumes, egg yolks, organ meats, blackstrap molasses, nuts, brown rice.

Vitamin C
Needed for healthy teeth and gums and connective tissue which holds cells together. Helps prevent varicose veins.

Citrus fruits and juices, broccoli, brussels sprouts, green peppers, parsley, rose hips, oregano, paprika, watercress.

Vitamin D
Necessary for proper absorption of calcium phosphate. Stores itself in the body.

Sunlight, enriched milk, fish oils, and liver oil.

Vitamin E
Controls the formation of fibrin, the blood-clotting element. Keeps the blood flowing smoothly. Helps maintain high oxygen.

Cold-pressed oils, eggs, wheat germ, organ meats, molasses, sweet potatoes, leafy greens, dessicated liver.

Vitamin K
Important for blood flow. Get plenty of Vitamin K during last trimester. Helps to clot blood. Pollution destroys Vitamin K in your body.

Alfalfa sprouts and tablets, dark leafy greens, soybeans, sunflower oil, egg yolks, blackstrap molasses, cauliflower.

Potassium
By activating many enzymes, it is essential for muscle contraction. Keeps sodium in balance in your system. Lack can cause edema (swelling).

Bananas, avocados, dates, elderberries, papayas, stewed prunes, legumes, dried apricots, sunflower seeds, lean meats, whole grains, vegetables.

Magnesium
Helps absorption of proteins and utilization of fats, carbohydrates, and enzymes. Keeps calcium in balance.

Whole grains, seafood, dark leafy greens, molasses, nuts, avocados, dates, dried apricots, bone meal.

Other Vitamins and Minerals
All fruits and vegetables.

The main thing I learned about nutrition during my pregnancy was to read the labels on the foods I bought. I was amazed to find out how many of my usual purchases contained unnecessary substances. Most of the foods had sugar or preservatives, neither of which my body or the baby needed to stay healthy. After all, enzymes have to work harder to digest foods that are "preserved." And sugar robbed my body of vital B vitamins, which were hard enough to put *into* my diet!

At the same time that I concentrated on eating properly, I was very careful about my weight. I knew that I should not gain more than 40 pounds. (More about weight gain later.)

It is important to choose foods from the four basic food groups. These are:

1. Meat, fish, and poultry
2. Fruits and vegetables
3. Dairy
4. Nuts, seeds, grains, and breads

I was primarily a vegetarian during my pregnancy, but I ate lots of eggs and cheese. It is possible to build a healthy body on a vegetarian diet. This chart of protein sources helped me choose foods high in protein. Let it help you too!

PROTEIN CHART

Food	Measure	Calories	Protein in Grams
Dairy			
Cottage cheese (lg. or sm. curd)	1 cup	235	31.0
Cottage cheese (dry or uncreamed)	1 cup	223	44.2
Whole milk	1 cup	159	8.5
Yogurt			
plain	1 cup	150	8.5
flavored	1 cup	280	12.0
Cheddar cheese	1 ounce	68	4.3
Brick cheese	1 ounce	103	6.2
Egg, 1 medium			
boiled, poached, or raw		79	7.6
scrambled		116	7.6

Food	Measure	Calories	Protein in Grams
Grains			
Barley	1 cup	782	18.0
Wheat germ	1 tbsp.	124	1.8
Brown rice	1 cup	748	14.0
Soy flour	1 cup	418	45.0
Fish			
Bass	1 pound	756	96.0
Bluefish	1 pound	720	118.0
Cod	1 pound	740	131.0
Flounder	1 pound	894	138.0
Haddock	1 pound	717	88.0
Halibut	1 pound	752	116.0
Salmon	1 pound	824	122.0
Swordfish	1 pound	764	129.0
Trout	1 pound	883	97.0
Tuna (canned)	1 pound	853	130.0
Meat			
Chuck, pot roasted	1 pound	1,481	117.0
Hamburger, lean	4 ounces	188	23.5
Heart, braised	1 pound	1,685	117.0
Kidney, braised	1 pound	1,142	149.0
Liver, fried	1 pound	1,052	120.0
Rump roast	1 pound	1,571	107.0
Round steak, lean	1 pound	856	141.0
Sirloin, T-bone, rib steak	1 pound	1,848	101.0
Turkey			
light meat	1 pound	797	149.0
dark meat	1 pound	920	136.0
Chicken, roasted	1 pound	1,314	114.0
Lamb shoulder	1 pound	1,264	145.0
Nuts and Berries			
Almonds	1 cup	765	26.0
Brazil nuts	1 cup	1,962	42.0
Peanuts with skins	1 cup	1,397	60.0
Pumpkin kernels	1 cup	1,271	67.0
Sesame seeds	1 cup	1,339	42.0
Sunflower seeds	1 cup	560	24.0
Walnuts	1 cup	651	15.0

(Continued on next page.)

Food	Measure	Calories	Protein in Grams
Beans			
Lima beans			
green, raw	1 cup	197	13.0
dry cooked	1 cup	265	15.7
Red kidney beans	1 cup	234	14.8
Garbanzo beans	1 cup	360	20.5
Lentils	1 cup	212	15.6
Split peas	1 cup	230	16.0
Soybeans	1 cup	260	22.0
Fruit			
Dried apricots	1 cup	390	7.5
Elderberries	1 cup	329	11.9
Papaya	1 large	156	2.4
Raisins	1 cup	462	4.0
Coconut, dried, unsweetened	3 ounces	662	7.2
Dried figs	3 ounces	274	4.3
Dried peaches	3 ounces	262	3.1
Vegetables			
Artichokes	1 medium	844	2.9
Asparagus	3 ounces	20	2.2
Beet greens	3 ounces	24	2.2
Black-eyed peas			
raw	3 ounces	108	21.8
dried	3 ounces	76	5.1
Broccoli	3 ounces	32	3.6
Cauliflower	3 ounces	27	2.7
Swiss chard			
raw	3 ounces	25	2.4
cooked	3 ounces	18	1.8
Collards, raw	3 ounces	45	4.8
Corn on the cob	1 cob	91	3.3
Kale, raw	3 ounces	53	6.0
Mustard greens, raw	3 ounces	31	3.0
Parsley, raw	3 ounces	44	3.6
Potato, baked	1 medium	93	2.6
Spinach, raw	3 ounces	26	3.2
Turnip greens, raw	3 ounces	28	3.0
Watercress, raw	3 ounces	19	2.2
Yam, baked	1 tuber	101	2.1

Women all over the world build healthy babies on all kinds of diets. If you prefer a meatless diet, discuss it with your doctor.

Throughout my pregnancy I ate as many foods as possible in their most natural state. In my search for whole foods, I relied heavily on the fresh produce section of the market. Nuts and seeds added sparkle to salads, sauces, and casseroles. You don't have to eat from all four food groups daily. You can spread the process out over two or three days. Your body takes a while to assimilate nutrients.

During my pregnancy I was interested to learn of a phenomenon we all have inside us: an amino acid pool. Amino acids are a part of proteins, and we need 22 different amino acids to complete a protein. Eight of these are not found in our system; we get them from the foods we eat. If, however, we eat foods that do not have complete proteins, our body will store the incomplete amino acids for up to twelve hours. If we eat a food that completes the group within that time, our bodies can utilize what they have stored to make a complete protein. Frances Lappe's *Diet for a Small Planet* and Ellen Ewald's *Recipes for a Small Planet* are both excellent books with easy recipes for combining foods to make the complete proteins we need.

It's fun and challenging to try to incorporate whole foods into your favorite recipes. With a little imagination, you can slip in a fresh fruit or vegetable with elegant results. Substitute honey, maple syrup, malt barley, or molasses for sugar. Parsley is a wonderfully rich source of iron. Used as a garnish, it can make even the simplest dish look fancy. And you can eat it, too. Whole grain crackers are a rich source of B vitamins and help you avoid the calories and bulk of bread. White breads are particularly hard on an intestinal tract that is being cramped by a growing baby. Foods that contain few nutrients not only waste space, but can rob your system of vital nutrients both you and your baby need.

When you fix meat dishes, try not to eat them with starchy vegetables like carrots or potatoes. Such combinations tend to cause the meat to digest slowly in your intestines, because your stomach starts to work on the starch first. This may cause heartburn. Make yourself a salad, broccoli, or other nonstarchy vegetable instead. As the baby grows, you will feel more comfortable eating smaller meals more frequently, so this is a perfect time to fix meals composed of one or two food items that combine well in your system.

Ligaments Affected by Pregnancy

Getting up suddenly during pregnancy may result in a twinge or cramp in your lower groin. I used to be zapped by a cramp, especially during the middle trimester. It was a relief to realize that the cramp was a sign the baby was growing. I tried to slow down my movements to avoid pulling on the ligament too harshly.

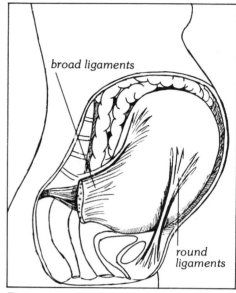

Figure 1-3.
The ligaments affected by pregnancy

Figure 1–3 will help you understand what those twinges are about. Notice the ligament in the front, the *round ligament*. It works like a pair of suspenders to support the uterus in a forward position. As the uterus grows, it stretches to accompany the increased size of the baby. It is this stretching process that causes twinging.

The other ligament that is affected by the baby's growth is your *broad ligament*, which attaches to the small of your back. The tug on your lower back from the baby's weight affects the broad ligament. This is one reason why proper muscle tone in your abdominal muscles and lower back is so important during pregnancy. You can increase circulation and lessen lower backaches and ligament twinges with proper exercise. (See the *Supermarket Walk* and *Pelvic Rocks* in Chapter 2.)

Varicose Veins

Varicose veins happen when the valve in the vein controlling the blood flow upward doesn't work properly. The blood flows backward, pools and distends the vein below the weak valve. They are common during pregnancy. Vitamin E can promote better circulation and thus help reduce the problem. If you have varicose veins, try not to sit in chairs for long periods of time. When you are at home or at friends', sit on the floor in tailor-sit position, or prop your back against the couch or wall with pillows. You might also lie on a couch on your side with your feet elevated. Five minutes on each side from time to time should help. Support hose offer some relief for those of you who are on your feet for long hours. Another helpful treatment is to wrap hot packs around your legs; use hot towels or washcloths.

Many times varicose veins are a problem because the weight of the baby restricts the flow of blood to the legs. Try exercises that move the baby forward or open the blood flow to your legs. *Pelvic Rocks* (see Chapter 2) move the baby forward and offer a better position for circulation. *Ankle Works* (see Chapter 2) also help to increase circulation in your legs.

Hemorrhoids

As we have seen, the baby's weight affects many parts of our anatomy. Hemorrhoids are a classic symptom of pregnancy. I didn't get them until I actually gave birth, but some women in my classes have lamented their presence during the last few months of their pregnancies. Putting a box next to the toilet for your feet to rest on, or squatting on the toilet, can help relieve some of the pressure to your rectum. Make sure your fluid intake is sufficient to help keep your stools soft.

Witch hazel is the traditional remedy for soothing itching hemorrhoids. Put some on a pad and apply gently to the irritated spot. The *Kegel Exercise* (see Chapter 2), which increases circulation and tones the whole pelvic floor, can offer relief. Sitz baths are a good friend for a sore bottom. In fact, pour a whole tub of hot water and treat yourself to a full bath. Use bubble bath (from natural sources— avoid too many synthetic chemicals) or a fragrance you enjoy, and make the experience an excuse for having some time to yourself. I enjoyed late night baths by candlelight.

Leg Cramps

Remember that during pregnancy nature considers the baby first. What she/he needs is taken from mother's nutritional supplies, and mother gets the leftovers. One nutrient that is in great demand from our system is calcium, which helps in the formation of bone and cell tissue. Unfortunately, the baby might take more than you are eating. If you experience leg cramps, a lack of calcium might be the problem. You can alleviate it simply by eating more foods that are high in calcium, for example, sesame seeds, carrots, or carrot juice, as well as raw dairy products. Homogenized or pasteurized dairy products are dead food and tend to be harder for the body to process. Your body assimilates a higher percentage of calcium when you eat raw dairy products (milk and cheeses that have not been homogenized and/or pasteurized).

You may also want to check that your salt intake is sufficient. For most Americans, it is. However, sometimes there is a salt deficiency related to leg cramps. One interesting dietary supplement is silica, which helps your body maintain a high level of calcium. Silica can be found in horsetail capsules. For women whose systems don't assimilate dairy products or don't benefit from calcium pills, this is an excellent source of "food" that helps your body create calcium from other chemicals present. I used them during my pregnancy, when I noticed my teeth were getting yellow. The calcium supplements weren't sufficient to meet my calcium needs. I found horsetail pills in a health food store, and within two weeks my teeth got whiter again.

One beautiful aspect of calcium is that it is nature's tranquilizer. I found an increase of calcium and horsetail intake calming on particularly frazzled days.

Leg cramps aren't always due to diet. The baby pressing down on your pelvis restricts circulation to your legs and feet and causes cramps. Try doing *Pelvic Rocks* and *Ankle Works* (see Chapter 2), or sleep with your legs slightly elevated. When you exercise, avoid stretching or pointing your foot too hard. This can cause instant cramping. If you do have a cramp, pressing your heel forward or stretching the muscles involved should relieve it. Sitting on the floor in tailor-sit position and loose clothes helps circulation.

Clothes

Dress during pregnancy is a subject close to my heart. Often the way you dress affects the way you feel about yourself. As you gain weight during your pregnancy and more and more of your clothes cease to fit, you can feel depressed. By viewing pregnancy as a time to find new and exciting clothes, however, you have a whole new realm of dressing available to you. I hated to go into maternity shops. The clothes they offered reminded me of a completely negative attitude about pregnancy from before our grandmothers' generation, when pregnancy was a hushed word. You hid it in clothes that didn't show your "condition." Have you ever noticed that when you wear loose or baggy clothing someone will say, "That makes you look pregnant," meaning ugly or unfashionable? Maternity shops too often have clothes which try to make the pregnant woman look like a sack of potatoes or a child. When you *do* buy standard maternity clothes, you might ask for 3-, 6-, and 9-month models—*not* sizes.

Luckily, there are ways of dressing open to you today that were not available to your mothers. You can get clothes that are comfortable and fashionable. Loose flowing skirts, overblouses, wraparound skirts or pants, or drawstring pants are relatively easy to find. You can also wear these after the baby is born. Long, flowing gowns or robes made out of an interesting fabric can transform you into a goddess. It's fun to experiment with ethnic and old-fashioned dress. I still have some of my maternity clothes, and they are wonderful. I call them my fat-thin wardrobe and wear them when I am a bit heavier or want to avoid wearing tight-fitting clothes around my middle. Leotards can also be bought in many different styles and colors. Since nylon doesn't breathe too well, I found that putting a mini-pad in the crotch helped prevent yeast. Cotton underwear is a must. Nylon panties block air flow, creating a lid effect which closes off your vagina. You need good circulation there to avoid yeast. You might even try going without underwear at home.

Sometimes a funny or decorative T-shirt can help you overcome the feeling of being fat or frumpy. You are building a baby, so of course you'll be gaining weight. But you still have the choice to look elegant, casual, or funky—whichever you choose!

Weight Gain and Water Retention

Weight gain during pregnancy varies from woman to woman depending on body type and diet. If you have a large frame, you might gain more weight to counterbalance the baby's weight. I gained 22 pounds during my pregnancy, and carried my baby out front. Other women might be round all over and gain up to 40 pounds. Gaining over 40 pounds adds too much weight for you to carry in addition to the baby.

There are many factors that influence where you distribute the weight you will gain. Your baby can weigh anywhere from 5 (just above premature weight) to 13 pounds. The average is 7 to 9 pounds. The placenta weighs almost 2 pounds. Amniotic fluid is around two and a half quarts of fluid weight. As noted previously, your breasts can gain a half to a pound in weight. Their swollen state under your armpit can sometimes cut off the blood flow to your hands, giving them a tingling or stiff sensation. *Single Arm Swings* or the *Milk Maid* (see Chapter 2) can improve the circulation problem.

33

Some of the weight gain during pregnancy is due to water retention. If you find yourself retaining too much fluid, eat natural diuretics like cucumbers, parsley, watermelon, and cranberry juice, and eat more easily digested proteins. Daily exercise, including ankle and wrist rotations, can help.

Sometimes fluid retention can be an indication that you need rest. One piece of advice I kept hearing over and over was to avoid taking soda preparations like Rolaids, baking soda, or Tums to relieve heartburn. They are very high in sodium, and unless your system is deficient, they tend to promote water retention, which is just what you *don't* want.

Heartburn

Weight gain is a healthy sign that your baby is growing. This growth pushes your uterus up, lifts your intestines, and tends to cramp other internal organs. In the case of your stomach, this shifting can result in heartburn. That's why your stomach does better with smaller but more frequent meals.

If you suffer from heartburn, avoid fatty, fried, or greasy foods. We've already seen that these cause gas. Try to identify any offending food source and eliminate it from your diet. (I love hot peppers, but my stomach didn't!) One woman told me she tried alfalfa tablets to ease heartburn and they worked within an hour. I was amazed to hear that something so simple could help her feel better. I wish I had known about them during my pregnancy. My solution was to eat papaya or take papaya tablets. Other women have sworn by yogurt and honey as a remedy. This is another one of those times you can get out the bottle of sparkling cider or bubbly water and pour yourself a glass.

THIRD TRIMESTER

Those Itchy Twitchy Feelings

I can remember nights when I wished that my legs could go out for a walk and let the rest of me go to sleep. They had more energy than I did. My solution was to do leg dances in bed. I would wave my legs in the air, use a bicycling motion, or draw letters in the air to music or my own sense of rhythm. This exercise helped me drift off to sleep.

Between having to use the toilet and putting up with a twitchy body, I didn't get much sleep during those final months. At first, naps were my best friend, but by the last two months, instead of wanting to sleep, I would read or think about what I would be like as a mother, about my labor and delivery, about what the baby would look like.

During my seventh month I began experiencing a hardening in my uterus. At first I thought the baby was stretching, but I noticed my uterus would stay hard for a while, then get soft again. My childbirth instructor told me that these were Braxton-Hicks contractions. My uterus was having dress rehearsals for the "real thing." These warm-up exercises continued for months. Whenever they happened, I would remind myself that my uterus was having a workout all on its own.

Shortness of Breath and Lightening

Those last few months were great postural reminders. If I slumped even for a minute, I found myself short of breath. As soon as I sat up straight, I could breathe more easily. Since growing babies take up a lot of room, they affect your diaphragm. Learning to do costal breathing (see Chapter 2) helped relieve my breathing difficulties. One other part of the pregnancy process helped tremendously—lightening. Lightening occurs when the baby's head drops or engages in your pelvic bones, in the inlet. When this happens, you can breathe more freely and

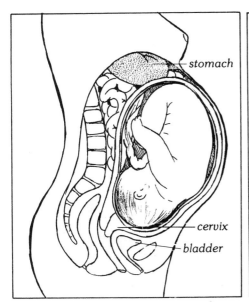

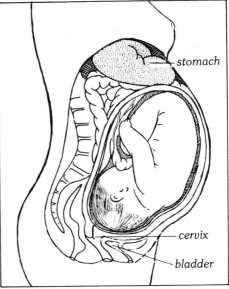

Figure 1-4.
Before lightening (at term—9 months)

Figure 1-5.
After lightening (at term—9 months)

eat more. You will also visit the toilet more often. Figures 1–4 and 1–5 both show a woman nine months pregnant; Figure 1–4 shows the body before lightening, Figure 1–5 after. Notice in Figure 1–4 that there is much less space for your stomach and lungs than in Figure 1–5. What you gain above you lose below.

When "lightening" strikes, you are in the home stretch. This phase of pregnancy is also called engagement and, with first babies, usually occurs a month to two weeks before the birth. From the second baby on, the baby can drop the day before the birth.

Lightening serves as useful warning. You may be a mother sooner than you expected. One practical piece of advice to make your last days of pregnancy as peaceful as possible is to tell everyone that you are due two weeks later than the predicted due date. That way you can avoid annoying phone calls asking if "it" has appeared. Only 5 percent of all babies arrive on their scheduled flight patterns. The other 95 percent come when they are ready, on the average of two weeks either side of the official due date.

Preparing Your Nipples for Breastfeeding

During the last month of my pregnancy I did all I could to toughen up my nipples. I wanted to breastfeed and had heard that babies are pretty rough on uninitiated nipples. I remember one day putting a friend's baby to my breast to see what it felt like. It hurt! I went right home and pulled, tweeked, brushed my nipples over and over with a dry washcloth. I was determined to get them in shape. By the time my daughter was born, they were ready.

Thinking Positively

Our thoughts and attitudes affect our entire beings. When we think positively, the world is a pleasanter place. Likewise, when we are down, or negative, the world seems to reflect that too. This is particularly true during pregnancy, when all our emotions are heightened. That's why your attitude toward your pregnancy can make the difference between feeling miserable or enjoying this special time.

I found that keeping a journal was a helpful way to turn problems into lessons. Sometimes when there was no one around to talk with I would write out the feelings I was experiencing. Then I would think of the positive thoughts, solutions, or alternatives to whatever my problem might be. Some days I couldn't change what was happening, but by making positive statements, I would come to feel better about myself. Relaxing, breathing, and acknowledging what I was feeling also helped me through days when I felt low or depressed. Pregnancy isn't all a bed of roses. But it *is* a time of constant challenge, a time to learn and grow.

The various complaints discussed in this chapter, taken together, may make pregnancy seem more like a pain than a joy. But the majority of your pregnancy can be delightful, full of new experiences and events. The more you know how to deal with the inevitable discomforts, the less anxious you will be, and the better equipped to live your daily life. Use the following summary as a check list:

Common Complaints and Suggested Remedies

Backaches
1. Be aware of your posture; avoid standing with your knees locked, stomach dropped forward, or back arched or swayed.
2. Do *Pelvic Rocks* to tone muscles and improve posture and circulation.
3. Avoid standing still for long periods of time, especially with your weight on one hip.
4. Be careful of how you bend and lift things. Never lift with your legs or back straight. See Chapter 2 for exercise hints on how to lift properly.
5. Wear flat or low-heeled shoes.
6. Apply hot pads to sore muscles, alternating with cold pads to promote circulation.
7. Massage the painful area with oils, such as olive, sesame and almond. This both alleviates aching and feeds your skin, for the oils are foods rich in vitamin E.
8. See the herb chart at the end of this chapter for herbs high in mineral content and rich in vitamin C.

Sore Breasts
1. Wear a well-fitted bra.
2. Apply a heating pad, or hot, wet towels.
3. Oil sore nipples with vitamin E or an oil rich in vitamin E such as wheat germ, olive, almond, sesame, or safflower oil.
4. See the herb chart at the end of the chapter for calming herbs.

Shortness of Breath
1. Sit up straight; improve general posture, creating more space for your lungs to breathe fully.

2. Do high costal (chest) breathing. (See Chapter 2.)
3. Remember that the condition will improve when the baby drops (lightening).

Constipation
1. Avoid straining while moving bowels.
2. Avoid taking laxatives; substitute diluted prune juice, fig juice, carrot juice, rhubarb juice, or stewed prunes.
3. Take two tablespoons of olive oil a day.
4. Eat high-fiber foods, like bran and salads.
5. Eat plenty of fresh and dried (soaked) fruits (except bananas).
6. Drink lots of fluids, especially water.
7. Get daily exercise, for instance, walking, swimming, or dancing.
8. Squat on the toilet, or put a box near the toilet for elevating your feet to facilitate evacuation.
9. See the herb chart at the end of the chapter for laxative herbs.

Fatigue
1. Get extra rest. Remember, your body is building a baby!
2. Avoid overdoing activities; take naps and rest breaks as often as you feel it is necessary. Your pacing will be different while you are pregnant.
3. Check for anemia. Eat foods rich in iron (see the nutrient chart on page 24).
4. If you are working, take more breaks. If possible, reduce working hours.
5. Eat foods rich in manganese such as whole grain cereals, egg yolks, green vegetables.
6. See the herb chart at the end of the chapter for high mineral herbs.

Gas
1. Identify the offending foods and avoid eating them (for now).
2. Lie down and do abdominal breathing; *The Turtle* exercise (see Chapter 2) can help.
3. Try *Pelvic Rocks* (See Chapter 2).
4. Check your food combinations. Simplify your meals.
5. Helpful herbs: anise or fennel seeds crushed and chewed, two or three drops of peppermint oil in a glass of water, chamomile.

Bleeding Gums
1. Increase vitamin C intake.

2. See your dentist.
3. See herb chart at the end of the chapter for herbs high in vitamin C.
4. Apply powdered white oak bark, myrrh, or a combination of slippery elm, golden seal, and white oak bark directly to the affected area.

Braxton-Hicks Contractions (hardening of the uterus)
1. Remember, these are generally good prelabor warm-ups for your muscles.
2. Do abdominal breathing.
3. Change activity and rest.
4. Keep in mind that these are good for the baby.
5. Consider the remote possibility of premature labor.
6. Helpful herbs: raspberry leaves, ginger root, and comfrey.

Headaches
1. Take a hot bath.
2. Relax, especially facial muscles, and rest.
3. Be cautious about aspirin and packaged remedies; they can adversely affect the baby.
4. Do *Head and Neck Rolls* (see Chapter 2).
5. If pain is persistent or severe, call your doctor.
6. Do alternate nostril breathing (see Chapter 2).
7. Press the bridge of your nose on either side with your thumbs, and rub firmly.
8. See herb chart at the end of the chapter for diuretic herbs (because sodium makes you retain water), and calming herbs.

Heartburn
1. Identify offending foods, watch food combining, and avoid all gassy, fried, or fatty foods.
2. Eat smaller and more frequent meals.
3. Don't eat close to bedtime, especially a big meal.
4. Eat papaya or take papaya tablets.
5. Eat yogurt and honey.
6. Drink sparkling cider or Perrier water.
7. Avoid soda preparations (they contain excessive sodium).
8. Avoid Rolaids or Tums (they contain 54 mg of sodium per tablet).
9. Helpful herbs: mint tea or chamomile tea, alfalfa tablets, oil of peppermint, elder flowers, marshmallow root, slippery elm, catnip.

Hemorrhoids
1. Put feet up on a small stool while sitting on toilet for bowel movement.
2. Do *Pelvic Rocks*.
3. Drink more fluids.
4. Take sitz baths.
5. Do lots of *Kegel Exercises* (see Chapter 2).
6. Apply witch hazel.
7. Helpful herbs: yellow dock tea; taro root (wild yam), grated, mixed with whole wheat flour, and applied as a poultice; a poultice of crushed chamomile leaves.

Itching Skin
1. Soothe your skin with oils, particularly wheat germ, almond, sesame, and safflower oil.
2. Increase your consumption of foods rich in vitamin E (see nutrient chart).
3. See herb chart at the end of this chapter for diuretic herbs.

Leg Cramps
1. Try *Pelvic Rocks* (see Chapter 2) to improve circulation, squatting and tailor sitting.
2. Sleep with your legs slightly elevated.
3. Avoid pointing your toes or stretching too hard.
4. Try not to cross legs and ankles.
5. Avoid constricting clothes.
6. Check to see if salt intake is adequate.
7. Try eating calcium-rich foods (see nutrient chart).
8. Try silica (from horsetail capsules).
9. Cut down on milk, or try raw milk.
10. Make sure you are getting enough exercise.
11. To stop cramping in progress: point your heel or stand on the affected leg, stretching cramped muscle.
12. See herb chart at the end of the chapter for herbs high in calcium.

Moodiness
1. Remember that this is a normal result of hormonal changes and extra blood and fluid, and it usually goes away.
2. Relax and talk with a friend.
3. Be nice to yourself!

4. See the herb chart at the end of the chapter for high-mineral herbs and calming herbs.

Nausea
1. Because this is often due to lowered blood sugar, eat small amounts of food often, especially protein and fruit (see protein chart on pages 26–28).
2. Eat dry crackers or toast in the morning before getting up.
3. Drink sparkling cider or Perrier water.
4. Get lots of rest.
5. Try remedies for an overstressed liver, such as vitamins B_6 and B_{12}.
6. See liver herbs and laxative herbs listed on the herb chart at the end of the chapter. Other helpful herbs are catnip, peppermint, basil, hops, lemon balm, and fresh ginger.

Pelvic Congestion
1. Do *Pelvic Rocks* (see Chapter 2).
2. Take hot baths.
3. Do *The Turtle* (see Chapter 2).

Sleeplessness
1. Be sure to get enough exercise.
2. Eliminate coffee, colas, black teas, and other caffeine-containing drinks from your diet.
3. Keep your emotional climate as serene as possible.
4. Sleep with extra pillows supporting your back and knees.
5. If you can't sleep, try reading, sewing, or finishing something you've put off doing before. Sleep when you are tired.
6. Try chamomile tea or warm milk.
7. See herb chart at the end of the chapter for calming herbs and high-calcium herbs.

Round Ligament, Stretching/Cramping
1. A sharp pain in the groin is often caused by cramping of the round ligament or a sudden growth spurt of the uterus. Do *Pelvic Rocks* (see Chapter 2).
2. Lean toward the cramped side as you would with a leg cramp until it eases. Rub gently.
3. Get up and lie down more slowly and gently.

Stretch Marks

1. Avoid rapid weight gains, especially near the last month.
2. Apply oils frequently to your skin, paying special attention to the abdomen, buttocks, thighs, and breasts. Oils rich in vitamin E such as wheat germ, sesame, almond, and safflower oil are particularly helpful.
3. Increase your consumption of foods containing vitamin E (see nutrient chart).

Vaginitis

1. Report to your doctor.
2. Eat yogurt and cottage cheese and add acidophilus to drinks.
3. Sit tailor fashion.
4. Wear cotton panties.
5. Take lots of warm baths.
6. Do *Kegel Exercises* (see Chapter 2) to increase circulation to the area.
7. Apply cottage cheese to a sanitary napkin and use as a poultice.
8. Helpful herbs: oat straw/comfrey douche, garlic suppositories behind cervix, the calming herbs listed on the herb chart at the end of the chapter.

Varicose Veins

1. Keep off your feet as much as possible.
2. Stay out of chairs; tailor-sit on the floor. If you must sit on a chair, put the sole of one foot against your other thigh (like half a tailor sit) resting gently on the chair.
3. Do *Pelvic Rocks* (see Chapter 2).
4. Lie on the couch on your side, with feet up on one arm or on pillows, for five minutes.
5. Do *Ankle Works* (see Chapter 2), *not* pointing toes. Repeat several times per day.
6. Increase vitamin E intake (see nutrient chart).
7. Wear support hose.
8. Put hot packs on legs.
9. Increase intake of foods high in vitamin C (see nutrient chart). Supplement your diet with lecithin and rutin (found in citrus fruits).
10. Helpful herbs: cayenne, herbs rich in vitamin C and vitamin E as listed on the herb chart at the end of the chapter.

Vomiting

1. Try to think of it as housecleaning, not an illness.
2. Sip fresh ginger root tea, sparkling cider, or bubbly water.

3. Helpful herbs: oil of peppermint and the calming herbs listed on the herb chart at the end of the chapter.

Water Retention
1. Get daily exercise but don't overdo.
2. Drink lots of liquids—water, juice (cranberry is good).
3. Eat more easily digested proteins.
4. Rest in bed if the problem is extreme.
5. Do ankle and wrist rotations.
6. Try natural diuretics like cucumbers, parsley, watermelon.
7. See herb chart at the end of the chapter for diuretic herbs.

Weight Gain
1. Understand that there is no set weight gain which can be applied to all women.
2. Eat a well-balanced diet including 65 to 75 grams of protein daily.
3. Avoid junk (empty) foods, fats, and sugars.
4. Get lots of exercise, walking, swimming, bicycling.
5. Helpful herbs: chickweed.

A Word About Herbs and Their Use

In this chapter I include herbs as an alternative for several different areas of relief. Herbs, like any plants, can be used to season foods (dillweed, basil, peppermint), can be drunk in tea form as a substitute for black teas or other caffeine drinks, or can be ground up and put into capsules to add certain vitamins or minerals to your diet. The growing popularity of herbs can be seen in the supermarkets, where some of the major tea companies are now marketing herb tea bags. For many years people thought asparagus was a suspicious weed to be avoided. Today asparagus is recognized as a delicacy. Herbs are food as well as a useful source of nutrition. For general information on herb use, I suggest you consult some of the books about them available at your local book store or health food store. The lists I have compiled here are meant to be used as a guide only, *not* a prescription. In all cases, start with a small dose and consult with a qualified person first.

The Most Commonly Used Herbs During Pregnancy

Alfalfa: High in vitamins A, D, E, and K. Helps digestion, is a source of protein, and can be eaten as tablets, sprouted, or drunk in teas.

Aniseed and *Fennel Seeds*: Both are aromatics, have a calming effect, help digestion, act as stimulants, increase milk flow. Crush the seeds to steep as a tea.

Capsicum (cayenne): Often thought of as a hot spice for foods, this herb is actually soothing to mucous membranes. A general system stimulant, it helps to balance circulation and works as a transporter bringing herbs where they are most needed in the body. It is best taken in capsules.

Catnip: Helps reduce heartburn, nausea, moodiness, and headaches due to its calming effects. It is also useful for sore breasts. Can be drunk as a tea or put in capsules.

Chamomile: Often planted in the gardens of Europe as a sedative; royalty would walk on it during their strolls to feel relaxed and calmed. A tonic to the gastrointestinal area, it reduces heartburn, gas, and bleeding gums. It also helps relieve backaches. Chamomile helps to cool the system down. The green part of the herb, crushed and made into a poultice, is useful for reducing hemorrhoids. Can be put in capsules and makes an excellent tea, especially pleasant after meals.

Ginger Root: Acts as an astringent and a transporter for bringing useful chemicals to the uterus; also has a calming effect helpful for reducing headaches and nausea. As a circulation stimulant it makes a strong-tasting tea.

Mint Family: Peppermint or spearmint are the most popular forms. They are relaxants, stimulants, and diuretics; they help digestion, relieve gas, and work best in tea combined with other herbs. Their leaves can be used in salads or with vegetable dishes as a spice.

Oat Straw: An herb rich in minerals, this is useful for vaginitis, and can be used as a douche. It has calming effect useful for backaches. When drunk as tea, steep for at least 15 minutes.

Parsley: High in iron and chlorophyl, this is a diuretic, helping to relieve congestion in the kidneys. Also it is good for backaches and reduces fatigue caused by anemia. Can be eaten raw or steeped and drunk as a tea.

Red Raspberry: The number one tea for uterine toning, it acts as an astringent, helps to tone pelvic girdle muscles, serves as a stimulant, aids digestion, helps to flush the system. It makes a tasty tea or can be put in capsules.

Valerian Root: This relaxant helps calm nerves, reduces headaches, helps counteract moodiness, soothes backaches, promotes sleep. It makes a very "earthy" tasting tea. It can be taken with hops and catnip in a capsule.

Yellow Dock: Another herb high in iron, it is great for reducing fatigue caused by anemia. It is a blood cleanser and a laxative, and it reduces hemorrhoids. It is quite strong tasting as a tea, sometimes easier to take in a capsule.

Warning: The following herbs should be taken only under the supervision and guidance of someone experienced in the use of herbs: bay leaves, blue or black cohosh, cotton root bark, ginseng, juniper berries, lobelia, mugwort, pennyroyal, peyote, rue, sage, squaw vine, tansy root, thyme, uva-ursi, western red cedar.

Although the above-listed herbs are not "dangerous," their preparation and combination for use by pregnant women require special knowledge.

HERB CATEGORIES

Calming Herbs: These herbs relax the system and work to soothe frazzled nerves.

catnip	lavender	red raspberry leaves
chamomile	lemon balm	skullcap
comfrey	mint family (peppermint,	squaw vine
hops	spearmint, etc.)	valerian root
horsetail	peach leaves	wheat grass juice

Diuretic Herbs: These herbs tend to increase the secretion of urine; they act promptly when taken on an empty stomach during the day.

alfalfa	horsetail	watercress
burdock root	marshmallow root	yellow yarrow leaves
cornsilk	parsley	yucca tablets
dandelion root		

Mineral-Rich Herbs, Calcium: This mineral is nature's tranquilizer and helps to relax the system. It is needed for the formation of good teeth and strong bones. During lactation, women require more calcium for nursing.

borage	dandelion root	kelp
chamomile	flaxseed	nettle
coltsfoot	horsetail	oat straw
comfrey		

45

Mineral-Rich Herbs, Potassium: This mineral is essential for muscle contractions, by activating many enzymes. It helps to keep your sodium in balance to prevent water retention.

alfalfa (sprouts too)	dandelion	parsley
borage	eyebright	peppermint
carrot leaves	kelp	watercress
chamomile flowers	mullein	wheat grass juice
coltsfoot	nettle leaves	yucca tablets
comfrey		

Mineral-Rich Herbs, General: All of these herbs have a high general mineral content.

blessed thistle	comfrey	parsley
borage	fenugreek	red raspberry leaves
burdock root	mullein	yellow dock root
chamomile	oat straw	

Laxatives: Like most herbs, these tend to work better when a few are mixed together in a tea or capsule. The juices should be diluted.
aniseeds
cascara sagrada
fennel seeds crushed, steeped
juice from figs, prunes, rhubarb
olive oil, 1–2 tablespoons a day
peach leaves
red raspberry plus alder buckthorn
senna plus mandrake root
wheat grass juice
white oak bark
yellow dock

Liver Herbs: These herbs help the liver repair and function fully. They tend to be high in iron and are slightly stronger tasting. You may want to put them in capsules.
dandelion root
fenugreek
licorice root

Vitamin C Herbs: This vitamin is needed for healthy teeth and gums. It tends to be destroyed by heat and cooking and therefore is better used in capsules. Because the body uses it quickly, a fresh supply must be provided daily.

capsicum	hibiscus	rose hips
chamomile	linden flowers	shepherd's purse
coltsfoot	paprika	violets
elder flowers	parsley	watercress

Vitamin E Herbs: Herbs rich in vitamin E cause dilation of blood vessels, permitting a fuller flow of blood to the heart. Vitamin E also helps to lower elevated blood pressure.

acerola	paprika
alfalfa	watercress
dandelion root	

Vitamin K Herbs: This herbal group helps the blood-clotting process, which is essential for a healthy birth.

alfalfa
shepherd's purse

2. *Prenatal exercises*

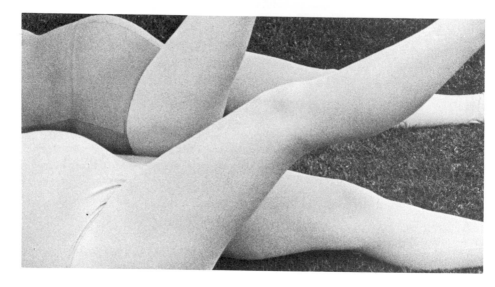

Pregnancy is an amazing process. With all of the changes your body is adjusting to, you may wonder, "Is exercise really safe for me?" Of course it is! Exercise increases your energy; it helps you prepare for labor and shortens your recovery time. It helps you look and feel your best.

Even if you have suffered a recent injury or had a miscarriage, you don't necessarily have to avoid exercise. However, you do have to keep your limitations in mind and you should check with your doctor first.

Since I was pregnant when I began teaching my prenatal exercise class, I had a deep personal interest in the movements I used. I questioned and analyzed each exercise as follows:

1. What muscles did it use?
2. How was it helping or otherwise affecting my pregnancy?
3. How would it help or affect my labor?

Whenever I experienced any strain or discomfort with an exercise or position, I would stop, relax, and try to figure out what had happened. Was I moving too quickly? Was I overdoing? Was my body too tight, or not strong enough? Then I would decide whether or not to continue.

It has taken me a number of years to develop the program presented here. The women in my classes have given me constructive feedback. Each woman's body is different. Some of my students haven't danced or exercised in years, and they express their concern about starting while pregnant. I reassure them, while reminding them that they need to listen to their bodies. They alone can sense when to move more slowly or stop.

I am often asked, "When should I start exercising?" My reply is, "As soon as you find out you are pregnant. If not then—right now!" It is never too early to start the exercise habit. Set aside a special time each day to devote to your body. This is a perfect way to nurture yourself and your baby.

Before my pregnancy, I had a history of lower back problems, pinched nerves, and a swayback. When I began exercising daily, my posture improved and my spine straightened. Whenever I felt a lower back pain, I would stop and do *Pelvic Rocks*. My back got stronger. Yours can too. Exercise will give you greater vitality and energy for mothering.

BASIC PRINCIPLES FOR MOVING THROUGH EACH DAY

Walking Gracefully

Exercise begins with posture, with everyday movements, with an awareness of how you feel inside your body. When you are walking, observe yourself. Don't change anything yet. Just observe. Become aware of what you are doing before you make *any* corrections or adjustments.

Begin by picturing in your mind your walking straight and tall. Let each breath bring fresh energy into your body. Let any tension in your shoulders "lift off." Take one hand and "dust" tired energy away. Brush your hand from your shoulder all the way down to your fingertips. Do it on both sides. Take a deep breath, then let it out long and slow. Now you are ready to walk tall and proud.

Many women carry their purses more on one shoulder than on the other. Try to give both sides of your body equal time. Better yet, get a small backpack and balance the weight in the middle of your back. This is especially helpful for long walks.

49

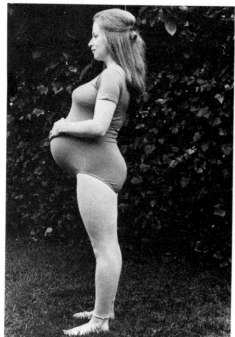
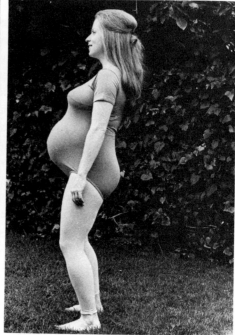

Not like this!   *Yes, this way!*

Make sure your shoes are low-heeled. Flat shoes are the best for your legs and spine, especially while you are pregnant. If you don't have flat shoes, invest in a pair. Your back is worth it.

Platform shoes are *out* for you during your pregnancy, except for walking very short distances. The same for high heels. They shorten your calf muscles and place a greater strain on your lower spine. In order to compensate for the off-balance position in which they place your body, you will be forced to sway your back. There are some very attractive flat-soled shoes on the market: Birkenstocks, Dr. Scholls, loafers, sandals, to mention a few. Be good to your feet and they will be good to your body.

What part of your feet do you walk on? The inside, or heels, or toes, or the middle? What about your knees? Are they locked or loose? How is your lower back placed? Long and lengthened, or short and swayed? Is one hip higher than the other? Is your abdomen lifted, or does it fall forward? Do your arms swing freely? Is your chest forward or back in relation to your abdomen? Is one shoulder higher than the other? (You can check this by noting whether one arm is longer than the other.) If you don't know the answers to these questions, have a friend watch you walk around the room and give you feedback. Go through this simple checklist: feet, knees, lower back, hips, abdomen, chest, shoulders, chin.

Note where these body parts are in relation to one another. You can avoid the "pregnant waddle." When you walk, let each leg swing forward easily. Feel the muscles under your buttocks gently push you forward. Lift up your abdominal muscles. Let your lower back lengthen. Feel your chest open and lift. Balance your shoulders. Let your arms swing freely. Let your chin gently pull back (not jutting out into space like a turtle peeking out of its shell). Feel the length of your neck as an extension of your whole spine.

This can be a relaxed, natural way to walk. You don't have to feel tense. You can feel lifted. Let your body "grow" into the proper alignment through your awareness of one part being on top of the part below it. It's as if you're stacking your bones. Walk with a sense of beauty and pride; remember, you are someone special—a pregnant woman.

Sitting Safely

Before sitting, stand with the back of your legs touching the seat. Then let your legs lower you slowly onto the seat. Never plop down!

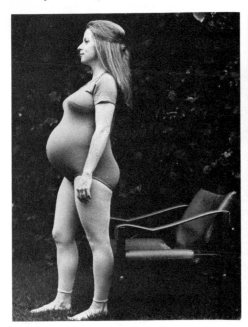 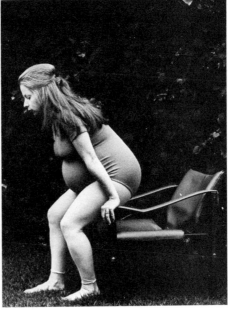

How to sit down correctly

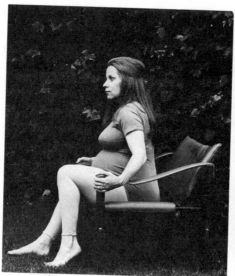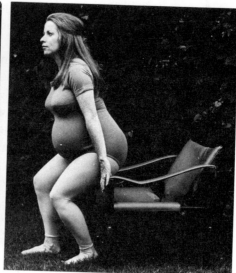

Getting up

A pregnant friend of mine once sat down too quickly on a seat that was lower than she had expected. She pulled her lower abdominal muscles, strained her round ligaments, and was very uncomfortable for several weeks. Get in the habit of thinking before you sit.

In general, when lowering or raising your body, let your legs help. To get up out of a soft couch or chair, slide forward to the edge of the seat, lean forward from your waist, and push down with your legs. This will help you rise slowly and gracefully. Pulling yourself straight up can be awkward and places an unnecessary strain on your abdominal muscles.

Climbing and Lifting

Stairs are a challenge to your legs. As you climb up, push from behind with the muscles under your buttocks. When you walk down the stairs, let your knees bend and lower your body.

When you need to bend over to pick up something, use your *legs*, not your back! Squat, or bend one knee, and lower your body. Avoid lifting with your back or legs straight. Instead, keep your knees bent and lift with your legs. When you lift any heavy objects, keep the center of the weight close to your body. This is

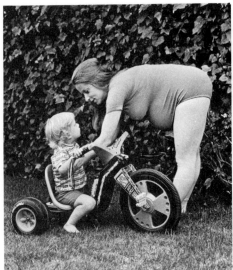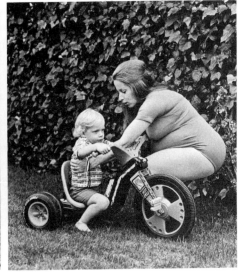

Please don't   **Try this instead**

a must for picking up small children. Your lower back will thank you for protecting it from strain.

All of this sounds simple, and it is. The challenge is to *remember* to put these principles to use. In the beginning, you will be establishing new patterns and so you may have to think consciously about moving in this new fashion. But by the third trimester, if you have practiced, you will be able to use these movements naturally. They will help you move through your pregnancy with greater comfort and ease.

DESIGNING YOUR PERSONAL EXERCISE PROGRAM

You don't have to do *all* the exercises shown in this chapter everyday. They are here to give you a wide variety to choose from. Change the order of the exercises you do each week. Make up different patterns. At the end of the chapter is one sample exercise pattern. You can pin it up on the wall as a gentle reminder to exercise each day. Vary your rhythms. Play different background music. Face in different directions when you exercise. Feel how each part of your body moves and flows.

Above all, enjoy the exercises. Experiment. There are many ways to move. Take each exercise as an example of how you *might* move, not how you *must* move. Some of the exercises have hints on how to "correctly" do the exercise. The reason for that is some of the movements are working on a specific set of muscles. If you move a different way, you might build a different set of muscles. That is all right also, but be aware of what you are doing. If you make a change, be conscious about what you are changing. If you think you need guidance, ask your doctor, an exercise teacher, or your childbirth educator.

In developing *your* exercise program, include at least one exercise from each of the following areas: head and neck; shoulders, chest and arms; back, abdomen, and waist; buttocks, pelvic floor, legs, and ankles; and breathing.

If you can, have someone read the exercises out loud to you, or put them on a cassette tape. For a list of available tapes, see the Resource Guide at the end of the book. Find a partner to exercise with you, preferably another pregnant woman. It adds to the fun. Some of the exercises in the chapter are especially designed for two.

Don't be discouraged if your body feels a bit tight at first. Keep moving and you will soon see and feel progress. Your body will let you know it is enjoying the attention.

As you exercise, remember:

○ Respect your body. Warm up slowly and build up the number of repetitions gradually.

○ Exercise gently. Avoid strain or stress. If you feel any pain, stop! Relax. Do some breathing exercises.

○ Limit the time you spend lying flat on your back. During the last three months of your pregnancy, do not lie on your back for more than five minutes. If you feel dizzy or light-headed, roll over to your side and bend your knees. Breathe gently.

○ Avoid exercises that cramp or suddenly shorten your lower back muscles, like the "bow" in yoga.

○ Sit up and lie down slowly. Avoid doing sit-ups, and don't use your abdominal muscles when lowering your back to the floor. To raise or lower your body, roll over onto your side and let your arms do the work.

○ Avoid bouncing. (It will not effectively stretch muscles.) Relax slowly and gently into stretches.

○ Never do *double* leg lifts. These can strain your lower back.

○ Avoid exercises that cramp the space for your uterus and constrict your

54

breathing—for example, putting your legs over your head or being upside down.
o Exercise on a surface that is firm and supportive—grass, carpet, or a foam mat (½ inch thick).
o Remember to breathe with all your movements!

BREATHING TIPS FOR EXERCISES

Strange as it may sound, most people forget to breathe when they exercise. We tend to hold our breath, or breathe very shallowly using only our upper chests. When you are exercising, think about the movements you are making. If the movement seems to be compressing your lungs, breathe out. Leg lifts, for example, require you to breathe out since you are compressing your abdominal muscles as you lift your leg. So does raising yourself or lifting an object. Conversely, when you are expanding your chest, breathe in. You will move through your day more efficiently when you follow your natural rhythms, expanding when you breathe in, contracting when you breathe out. Experiment with your own breathing patterns as you exercise. See what works best for you.

Proper breathing is an important ingredient in a successful labor. Childbirth classes teach various breathing techniques. The two that will be most helpful during pregnancy *and* labor are abdominal and costal breathing. Abdominal breathing is a long, low, deep breath that pushes your diaphragm down and pushes your abdominal wall out. (See the Exercise Section for details.) Costal breathing is a higher, chest-centered breath. It presses the rib cage out to the side, rather than extending your abdomen out.

Other techniques designed to increase your breathing repertoire are included in the Exercise Section. Practice them now, building up the endurance you will need later. When your labor time comes, follow your instincts. As long as you do not tense or try to hold your breath (unless you are pushing), you will breathe as you need to.

During my labor, I used abdominal breathing for almost the entire time. But I was glad that I had other techniques in my repertoire; it gave me a feeling of confidence. The same will be true for you. Learn to breathe as you need, when you need. If you want to change your rhythm, style, or focus, do it. You'll know what works for you.

Beginning with breathing techniques, the following exercises are arranged to follow each other in a smooth, flowing form. Read the directions out loud first or follow a tape. (See the Resource Guide.) Now let's begin. This is a dance for you and your baby—a baby dance.

BREATHING EXERCISES

Abdominal Breathing

Picture your abdomen as an empty glass. As you draw in air, you will pretend it is water, filling the glass from bottom to top. This allows your abdomen to "rise up" off your uterus. As you let air out, the glass empties from the top to the bottom. This lowers your abdomen back onto your uterus.

Now, sit with your legs crossed, and imagine your glass filling as you breathe in, letting your abdomen expand out.

Exhale, and let your abdomen push gently inward.

When you first practice this exercise, place your hand on your abdomen. As you inhale, push gently out and feel your hand lift. As you exhale, let your hand lower slowly as you press in. Each time you practice, lengthen your inhalation and exhalation. Picture your spine as a channel. Inhale and draw energy up your spine. Exhale and push tension or negative energy down and out your spine.

The name for this exercise is misleading. You aren't "breathing" with your abdomen, you are lowering your diaphragm as you inhale. This action pushes down on your intestines, which are in a very limited space. This makes it appear that you are pushing your *abdomen* in and out. The main focus is on relaxing the abdomen so you can allow your chest to rest. You will be breathing more deeply and fully.

During my pregnancy this breathing helped me through tiring days. It gave me a skill I could use to help relax. I would sit down for five minutes and focus on my breathing. Without fail, I would get up having more energy, feeling calmer, and being ready to go on with my day.

When I went into labor, I used this breathing for almost the entire time, about twelve hours. Breathing slowly and fully in this way enabled me to "ride" my contractions. Between contractions, I was able to use my breathing to let go of any tight areas and to relax.

Costal Breathing

Put your hands on your ribs. Inhale and push your hands out.

Exhale and feel your ribs come together, compressing the air out gently.

By your last trimester you may find it harder to breathe, especially when you are sitting. Some days I wanted to arch up and back just to get enough space to breathe. I decided there had to be another way of breathing that would bring in more oxygen. As there wasn't much room in front, I focused on my back and on the sides of my rib cage. I thought, "If I breathe out to the sides and expand my rib cage, I will be able to breathe more fully." I tried it and the breath worked. I also felt more space between my shoulder blades. My back opened and relaxed, releasing tension I had stored there.

This breathing pattern is best suited for pregnancy. However, you could use it during labor to relax your diaphragm and stretch the muscles around your rib cage. Think of it as a tool. If you need it, use it.

Candle-Blowing Breath and Panting

Candle-blowing breath
Imagine a large cake in front of you topped with 200 lit candles. You are going to blow them all out. One at a time.

Take a cleansing breath: inhale through your nose, hold, and exhale through your mouth. Now inhale and blow out seven times, letting your cheeks puff out and relaxing your jaw.

Stop, and slowly inhale. Let the air out very slowly. Repeat this breath cycle until you have blown out all your candles.

The main difference between candle-blowing breath and panting is the position of your mouth and jaw. Both breathing patterns are used to prevent pushing in labor.

Panting
Let your tongue hang loose in your mouth. Pant slowly like a dog on a hot day. Now try the candle-blowing breath again: Decide which one is more comfortable for you, and use that one. The main concern here is to relax your jaw, focus on your breath going out, and concentrate on your breathing. Let yourself breathe slowly and rhythmically to avoid hyperventilating.

Both of the above techniques are valuable additions to your breath repertoire.

There are two specific times during labor when you might want to use them:
when you feel the urge to push before you are fully dilated;
when your baby's head is crowning and you want to avoid pushing in order to minimize tearing (and the need for an episiotomy, an incision in the tissues between the vagina and the rectum).

However, do NOT use any type of rapid breathing for long periods of time. Keep your breathing slow!

Alternate Nostril Breathing

Sit down. Take the index finger of your right hand and cover your left nostril. Inhale through your right nostril.

Close your right nostril with the thumb of your right hand. Remove your index finger and exhale through your left nostril.

Inhale through your left nostril, then close the left nostril with your index finger. Remove your thumb and exhale through your right nostril.

Continue breathing through alternate nostrils. Focusing your breath on one side of your nose at a time utilizes the different centers in your brain, helping to balance right and left brain centers.

I did not find this breathing pattern useful for labor, but I did find it an invaluable tool during my pregnancy. It helped clear my thoughts, removed my headaches, and made me feel calmer. Some of the women tell me that it clears their nasal passages and helps them breathe better.

BODY MOVEMENTS

Kegel Exercise *pelvic floor*

In this exercise you are working on your vaginal muscles, those muscles which can be felt when you stop the flow during urination. To exercise these muscles, using imagery:

Place your hand on your lower abdomen. Your hand can help you feel whether or not you are tensing your abdominal muscles. You should avoid tightening those muscles. Remember to slowly contract and relax your vaginal muscles only. You will need to relax those muscles to help your baby out; you will need to tense them to help you feel where they are, and to tone them. You want to isolate and use only the muscles in your pelvic floor.

Imagine the floor of your pelvis to be an elevator. You will be going up slowly to the fourth floor. Contract your vaginal muscles gradually. Count slowly from one to four as you tighten a bit for each floor.

Pause. Now you have fully tightened your vaginal muscles, and you are on the fourth floor.

Take the elevator back down, one floor at a time. Let your pelvic floor muscles relax gradually until you reach the ground floor. Go one level further down, into the basement. Focus on relaxing your vaginal muscles even more.

This is one of the most important exercises for childbirth, sexual pleasure, and the prevention of prolapsed organs later in life. This is when the pelvic organs drop down in the vagina due to weak pelvic floor muscles. You are helping the circulation in your vaginal canal; you are promoting an awareness of the place from which your baby will emerge; and you are toning the floor of your pelvis for a faster recovery.

An ideal time to practice is during intercourse. You might call this a sex-ercise. You can both enjoy this exercise time together.

Kegels must be done every day—100 times. You can practice them everywhere: while doing dishes, walking, standing in lines, talking on the phone, taking a bath. One lady used to tell how long the traffic signals were on the way to class by the number of *Kegels* she had done waiting for them to turn green!

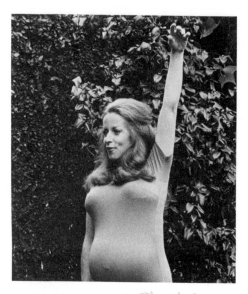

Single Arm Swings

Stand with your feet parallel, approximately hip-width apart. Take a cleansing breath: inhale through your nose, hold, and exhale through your mouth.

Inhale as you swing one arm forward in four continuous circles.

Pause, and exhale as you reverse direction of the circles. Alternate sides.

This exercise relaxes the muscles feeding into your neck, upper back, and shoulders.

Let your arm swing easily, like a propeller winding up. As your breath capacity increases, you will be able to inhale and exhale longer, making more arm circles in each direction with each inhalation. When inhaling, imagine you are drawing energy in. With each exhalation, feel the tension flowing out through your fingertips.

Your pregnancy creates a need for more oxygen in your system, both for your baby and for you. Allow the air to come into your body easily. Don't force it. Let the momentum of the movement create the circle.

By the end of your pregnancy, your body will be carrying 25 to 45 percent more fluid, creating more tension than usual. One of our chronic tension areas is the neck and shoulders. Easy circles with your arms can loosen up some of that tension and prevent headaches. So swing energy in and send tension out. Begin your day fresh and alert.

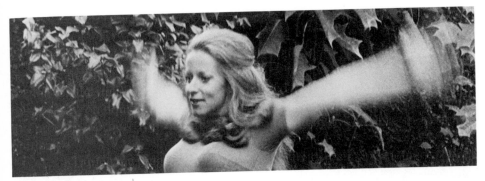

Milkmaid sh. ch. arms.

Stand with your feet parallel, approximately tummy-width apart. Take a cleansing breath: inhale through your nose, hold, and exhale through your mouth.

Hold your arms straight out to the sides, shoulder high, palms facing forward. As you draw five large circles to the sides, inhale with short, sniffing breaths, one for each circle.

Now make five large circles in the opposite direction. Exhale with short sniffs, one for each circle, as though you were blowing your nose.

This exercise strengthens your shoulders and upper back muscles. Also, by placing your palms forward, you help to tone your pectoral muscles.

Now put one hand above your opposite breast, fingers pointing toward your armpit. Circle your outstretched arm with your palm facing forward. Do the same with your palm toward the floor. Do you feel a difference? When your palm is forward, you engage your pectoral muscle. This muscle helps to support your breasts, which have already begun to enlarge.

Here is another opportunity to let tension go and draw energy in. As you inhale, draw energy in through your arms. As you exhale, let your shoulder tension flow through your arms and out your fingertips. Let your movement be big and bold. Feel the power in your whole upper body.

You may notice that you tend to take shallow breaths, filling only your upper chest. You need more air. Your baby receives its oxygen from your blood through the placenta. As you breathe in, the blood passing through your lungs exchanges carbon dioxide for oxygen. The oxygen gets passed on through your blood to your baby. Deeper, fuller breathing increases the oxygen content in your blood and so gives more to your baby.

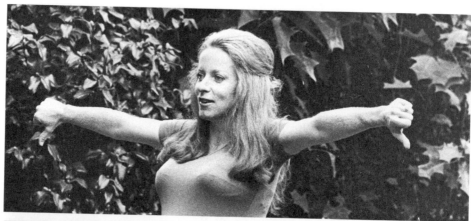

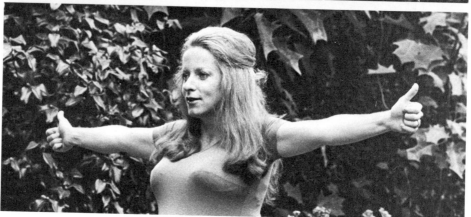

Thumbs Down Sh Ch ams

Stand with your feet parallel, tummy-width apart, and stretch your arms out to the side.

Make a fist, leaving your thumb sticking out; point your thumbs toward the floor.

Rotate your arms so that your thumbs point back up toward the ceiling. Continue turning your thumbs up and down.

While you rotate your arms, exhale and inhale through your nose, with short bursts, as if you were blowing out a candle with your nose.

Increase your breath rate slowly, then gradually decrease it.

Take a deep cleansing breath, fold your arms over your chest, and relax.

Rotating your hand tones your underarm area, your triceps. The breathing pattern used here, called the "breath-of-fire," helps to tone your abdominal muscles, which energetically push in when you exhale. It also strengthens the intercostal muscles around your rib cage by pressing your ribs together forcefully as you exhale.

You should feel plenty of muscular action in your arms as you do this exercise. As a result you'll have stronger arms to lift and carry your baby, and you'll avoid underarm flab.

Be careful not to overdo the breath pattern. You can easily hyperventilate and might find yourself getting dizzy. This occurs when your brain receives too much oxygen, depleting the carbon dioxide in your system. You need a balance of oxygen and carbon dioxide to breathe properly. Find your limit. Let your breathing speed up and slow down gradually. At the end of each set, exhale long and slowly.

After practicing this exercise for a while, you will learn how to control your breathing rate. During labor this will help you maintain a relaxed, comfortable breathing pace.

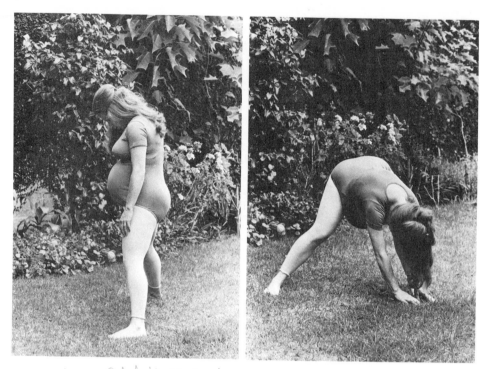

Raggedy Ann Abd, Waist, Back

Stand with your feet parallel, approximately tummy-width apart. Imagine you are a puppet. Now cut the strings that hold up your head, your neck, your shoulders, your ribs, your waist, and your hips.

Let your body give in to gravity. Now, bend and straighten your knees. Sway gently from side to side, from the base of your spine, like a large elephant's trunk. As you sway toward a knee, bend it. Straighten it as you sway away.

Stop swaying. Let your body hang quietly, bend your knees, and put one hand on each leg. Slowly draw your hands up the front of your body, as you straighten up slowly, all the way over your head, taking as many breaths as you need. (Be sure to come up very slowly to avoid dizziness.) With a sigh, lower your arms down to your side.

You are stretching the muscles in the back of your legs and lower back.

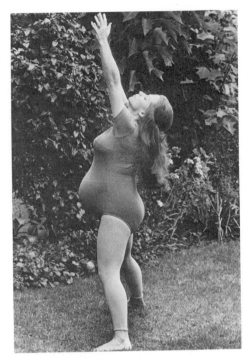

Allow yourself to relax into this exercise. It is one of the few moments you will spend upside down while pregnant. Enjoy the sensation of stretching. Feel the blood flowing freely to your head. You are increasing circulation to your brain and bringing roses to your cheeks.

Remember to bend your knees when you slowly straighten your back. This action helps bring your abdominal muscles into use, relieving your lower back muscles from doing all the lifting.

The weight of the baby pressing down constantly on the blood supply to your legs tends to reduce circulation. In this exercise you let the baby fall forward and thus increase the circulation to your legs. Increased blood flow (and vitamin E) also prevent varicose veins.

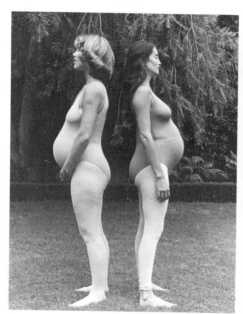 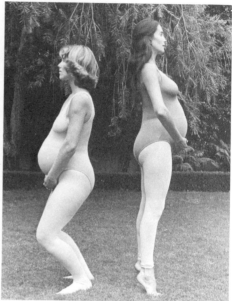

Elevator ~~Back Legs, Ankles~~

Stand with your feet parallel and tummy-width apart.

Inhale as you slowly bend your knees, keeping your heels on the ground. Lower yourself as far as you can with your back straight and long.

Straighten your knees gently.

Exhale as you rise up onto the balls of your feet.

Slowly lower your heels back to the ground as you inhale.

This exercise strengthens your ankles, stretches your calf muscles, and builds up the muscles in your lower leg. It also helps the circulation to your feet.

Your posture is important when you do this exercise. You are heavier in front now and will need to make adjustments to compensate for the added weight. Before you start, feel your feet. Is your weight in the middle of your foot? Rock forward and back gently until you feel your weight in the center.

Notice your ankles as you do the exercise. If they are doing a lot of rolling in and out, stop. Go up and down only as far as you can without any wobbling. In the beginning you might hold onto a doorknob or a ledge with one hand to help keep your balance.

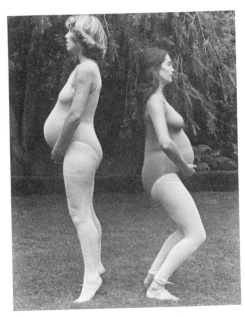

When you bend your knees, let them go over your toes. Look down. Do your knees cover your big toe when they are bent? If so, you're doing the movement correctly. If you can see your big toe, inside or outside of your knee, you need to use your inner thigh muscles more to guide your knee.

Also, when bending your knees, be careful not to slump your chest forward. Let your breathing help you. As you bend and inhale, fill your chest with air. Now feel your torso lengthening. When you rise up on the balls of your feet, watch that your back doesn't arch. Push your breath out and raise your body effortlessly. Your baby will enjoy the ride too!

This is another exercise that, done daily, improves your circulation and reduces the occurrence of varicose veins. If you notice any puffiness around your ankles, this exercise can help to reduce that swelling. It may also be a sign that you need to rest more during your busy day. Remember, you are building a baby!

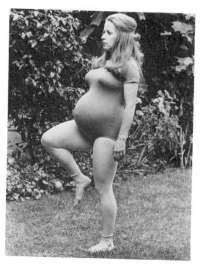

Supermarket Walk *Back, Abd & Waist, Legs,*

Walk forward. As you step, swing your leg forward and lift your knee, raising it toward your chest. As you make a circular path with your knee, be sure your foot is relaxed. Swing your foot back to the ground.

Continue walking, lifting alternate knees. Be sure to stand straight and tall as you walk.

This high prancing walk helps tone and strengthen your round ligament, which supports your uterus in the front like suspenders. It also helps to tone your thigh and abdominal muscles.

The name for this exercise came to me one day in class. We were prancing around the room, and suddenly my imagination transported us all to a supermarket. There we were, strutting down the aisles with our shopping baskets, feeling so proud to be pregnant!

As your uterus goes through growth spurts, you may feel a cramp or sharp pain in your lower abdomen. We have already discussed how this can occur when you stand or sit too quickly. Your body is probably telling you to slow down. Or the discomfort may be healthy proof that your baby is growing, stretching your uterus, pulling on your round ligaments. The supermarket walk tones your round ligament and helps give it more elasticity. This prevents some of the sharp pains that can occur if it is not toned when it stretches. However, if the pain persists, call your doctor.

68

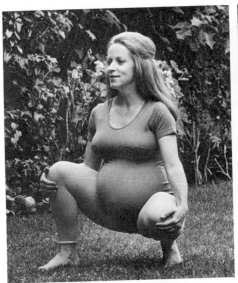 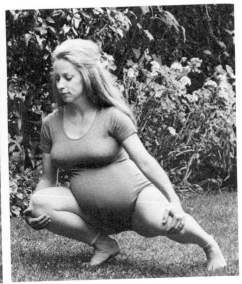

Monkey Walk <u>Back, Legs, Ankles,</u>

Stand with your feet tummy-width apart and take a cleansing breath.

Lower into a squatting position and walk around, in a wide circle. Let your arms hang down in front of your feet helping you walk forward.

This exercise strengthens your thighs and ankles and stretches your lower back.

True, this is not the most graceful exercise, but it's good for you. GI's who do it in basic training call it the duck walk. It always makes me feel like a monkey. Be sure to use your arms if you need them for balance. Get the whole family monkey walking.

We are among the few mammals to carry our pregnancies in a vertical position. Most animals have it easier because they are on all fours. The *Monkey Walk* lowers your center of gravity and gives your legs a good workout. It also helps to prevent varicose veins by strengthening your leg muscles and improving circulation.

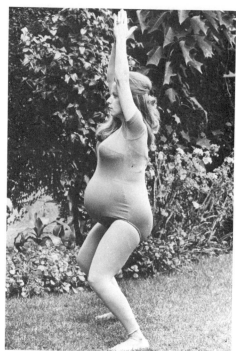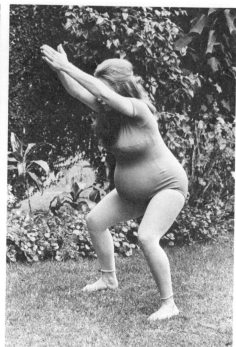

Squatting Breath _Ankles, Pelvic Floor, Legs, Back_

Stand with your toes pointing out and your feet approximately tummy-width apart. Take a cleansing breath.

Inhale and bring your palms together over your head.

Lean forward, bending at the hips. Exhale as you bend your knees, keeping your feet as parallel as possible, with your weight in the center of your foot. Keep your heels on the ground if possible.

Inhale, keep your knees bent, put your hands on your legs, and draw them up the front of your body above your head.

Let yourself sigh as you exhale. Let your arms float down to your sides. Straighten your knees gently.

Squatting stretches your calves and strengthens your ankles and lower leg muscles. It also stretches and tones your perineum (the area between your vagina and rectum).

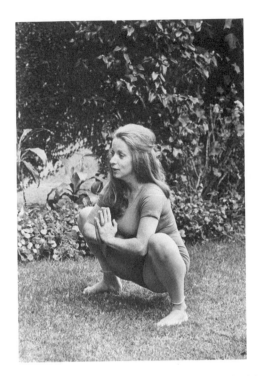

If you have any problem squatting, hold onto a door by both knobs. This has helped many women in my classes. Have your feet tummy-width apart and lower your body slowly to the floor. Keep your heels on the ground. When you lift up, keep your back long and straight. Let your arms help you up.

When you move away from the door, if your heels still don't touch the floor, be patient. It took me a few years to successfully touch the ground with my heels. It will happen for you, too, with practice.

Squatting lets your uterus gently fall forward, giving your intestines more room. It also helps prevent hemorrhoids.

This exercise is a good preparation for playing with your child later on. You can squat to be on his/her level more easily. You can pick up toys, and avoid straining your lower back when you lift your baby.

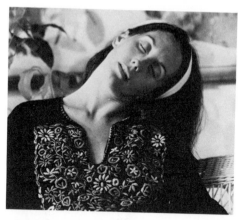

Head and Neck Rolls *Head & Neck, Back*

Sit with your legs crossed (tailor-sit).

Let your chin drop to your chest and roll your head around slowly, making a full circle.

Relax your shoulders, sit tall and quietly. Reverse direction.

Sitting in this tailor-sit position helps open your inner thighs and strengthens your back muscles. At the same time, the circular movement with your head relaxes the tension in your neck.

Your upper back muscles help to support almost twelve pounds of head. Treat your neck with this exercise. "Roll" tension off your neck. Visualize a beam of bright light shining out of the top of your head. This helps to keep your neck long and avoid any "crunching" (shortening of any part of your neck).

Our way of sitting, primarily in chairs, couches, and other supportive furniture, has deprived us of the use of our back muscles. We need to strengthen them. When you sit, try to use the tailor-sit position, even when you are sitting in a chair. Never sit with one leg crossed over the other. Yes, I know we are trained to sit that way; however, it cuts off the circulation to the legs and lower back. Our fashions, which allow us the luxury of loose, flowing skirts and pants, give us the freedom to sit with our legs apart, covered by our clothes.

By strengthening your back and stretching your inner thighs, you can sustain your energy while pushing during childbirth. This strength will also help you to recover faster. And with a strong back, you will be able to carry your baby more easily.

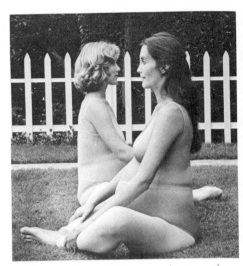 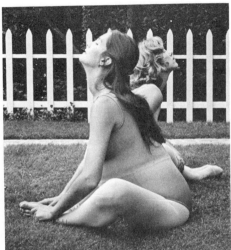

The Wave: Soul Version *Head & Neck, Back, Abd & Waist, Legs*

Sit, placing the bottoms of your feet together at a comfortable distance from your groin.

Lean forward, leading with your chin, and exhale.

Inhale, while tucking your chin into your chest and curling your spine back up to a sitting position.

Keep repeating with a circular, wavelike motion. Relax your arms and shoulders; let them ride the wave.

This exercise stretches your spine, the back of your legs, and your neck. The neck motion also stimulates your thyroid and parathyroid glands, helping assimilation of nutrients for proper hormonal balance.

While I was pregnant, I wanted exercises to flow and feel light. The image of the wave helped me create a seaside setting in my mind. Other women told me they felt graceful doing this exercise. By visualizing sand and sea, you can create your own pleasant environment and reinforce good habits for labor.

Before my labor I had discussed with my coach what images helped relax me. We practiced, and during labor he whispered images of water flowing around and through my body. It helped lower my tension level and lighten the contractions.

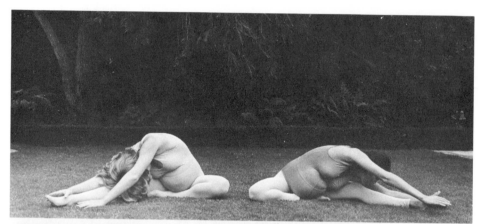

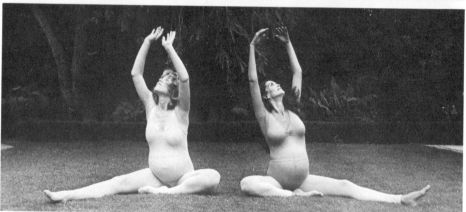

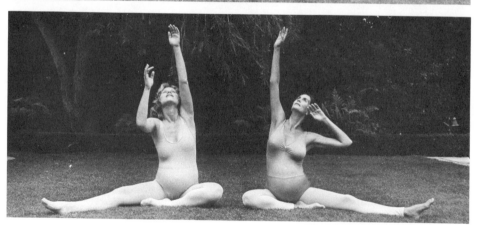

The Wave: Open Version *Head & Neck, Back, Legs, Abd & Waist*

Sh. Ch & arms
Sit; extend one leg to the side and place your other foot against your upper thigh.

Extend your arms overhead and inhale as you stretch up for something just out of your reach. Twist toward your extended leg, reach out with your hands, and exhale as you lean forward, leading with your chin.

Let your chin drop back toward your chest, curl your spine back to a sitting position, let your hands slide back up your legs easily with a circular, wavelike motion of your spine and arms. Do several waves before you extend your other leg and repeat on the other side.

This exercise stretches the back of your legs and your lower back. It also increases circulation to your legs.

Allow your back to relax as you imagine waves rolling over your spine. The wave can also let you feel the length along the front of your body, when your chin stretches forward.

As you reach forward, stop and stay arched over your leg. Allow the weight of your body to help you hang forward. Feel the back of your legs. The stretching "tenderness" you feel provides you with a wonderful opportunity to practice relaxing into an uncomfortable sensation. Imagine you are having a contraction. Breathe and let your body surrender into the stretch. During labor, when your cervix is opening, your best tool is breathing and accepting the process. Know that by relaxing you will ease your labor. Practice now—you will be glad you did.

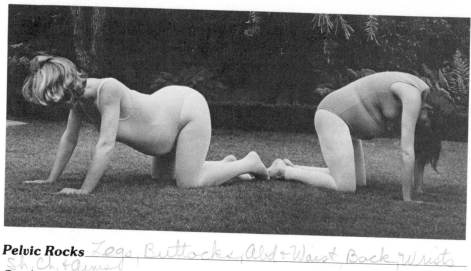

Pelvic Rocks *Legs, Buttocks, Abd & Waist, Back, Wrists, Sh, Ch, & Arms*

Get down on your hands and knees, knees slightly apart. Make sure your arms fall straight from your shoulders and your legs fall straight from your hips.

Tuck your pelvis under and forward, pull up your abdominal muscles, push with the muscles under your buttocks.

Let your tummy drop gently, relax and sway your back into a gentle curve. Continue the rocking action. Sway and tuck, sway and tuck. Be sure to isolate your lower back muscles and avoid arching your upper back.

Pelvic rocks strengthen your lower back, your wrists, your abdominal muscles, and your upper leg muscles. They also let your baby fall forward, allowing more space for your intestines. This exercise also improves circulation in your legs, thus preventing varicose veins.

When you rock your pelvis, feel the muscles under your buttocks pushing forward. This pushing helps to tone those muscles as well. Allow yourself to relax and flow with a gentle rocking motion. Let your buttocks tuck only as far as you need to make your back flat, not arched. Remember that you want to isolate your lower back muscles.

This exercise is both a key to a comfortable pregnancy and a useful lifetime tool. Do it often. Whenever you have back pains, stop and find a position in which you can do pelvic rocks. You can even do them standing. Hold onto a counter or a shelf. Arch your back, then tuck your buttocks under. Rock your hips gently forward and back. Or you can try them when you sit in a chair. Tip your pelvis forward, then press the small of your back against the chair back. These are essentially the same movements that you did on all fours. Your lower back will thank you.

If, during labor, you have back labor or any pains in your back, get in the pelvic rock position. You may want to rock between contractions. I had back labor for six hours and I used this position to relieve some of the intensity I experienced. My daughter's head was transverse, sideways, when I began pushing. Resting on all fours, coupled with rocking my hips from side to side, helped to rotate her head to an anterior position, one of the most common positions in which the fetal head emerges.

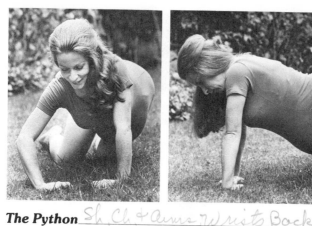
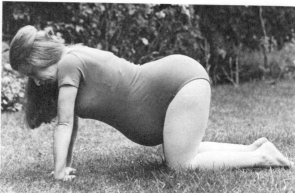

The Python Sh Ch & arms Wrists Back

On your hands and knees, roll your rib cage around as if your ribs are inside a barrel.

Arch your back, and push your ribs to one side. Sway your back gently, bending your elbows. Push your ribs to the other side.

Allow the movement to be continuous and smooth. Let the circles massage your shoulder blades.

This exercise works on your middle back and rib cage, strengthening and toning the muscles.

Let yourself luxuriate in the rolling sensation. This part of your back stores a lot of tension that can be relieved by rotation. Massage also helps, and I prefer that any day, but when I'm alone this exercise really helps.

Sitting, relaxing, and pushing all require good tone in your middle back. After your baby is born, holding and carrying will require strength there too. Build it now.

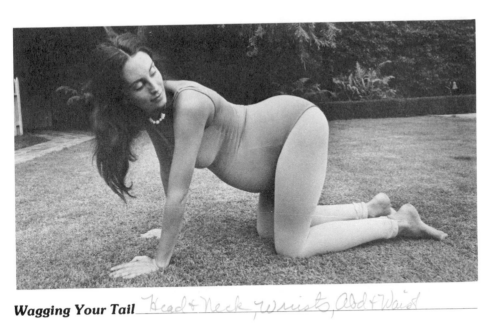

Wagging Your Tail Head & Neck, Wrists, Abd & Waist

Visualize yourself with a tail. It can be any size, color, and shape you choose.

Inhale and look at your tail over one shoulder. Exhale as you return to facing forward. Repeat on the other side.

"Wagging" is good for your waistline, which is hiding in there somewhere. It also helps tone the muscles that wrap around your torso.

During labor you will want the muscles that support your torso to be in good tone to help bear down and push your baby out. It is also nice to remember that your waist *will* return after the birth.

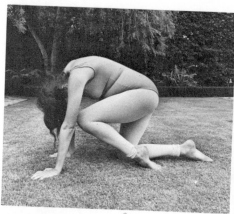 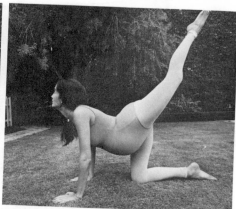

Bucking Bronco *Legs, Buttocks, Back, Wrists, Sh, Ch + arms*
Head + neck

On your hands and knees, exhale and swing one knee forward, toward your chin.

Inhale as you gently swing your leg back and turn up your eyes, lifting your head. Swing the other leg, and keep alternating sides.

Gentle kicking and arching stretch and strengthen your lower back and loosen your hip joint.

Let your leg swing freely as you bring your knee toward your chin. If you have any difficulty, try swinging your arm to feel the sensation of an easy, pendulum-like motion. Then go back and try it on all fours with your leg.

As much as I loved *Pelvic Rocks*, I wanted another exercise for strengthening my lower back. As my baby grew larger, it was obviously harder to swing my leg as high or as close to my chin, so I lessened the range and thrust of the swing to avoid strain.

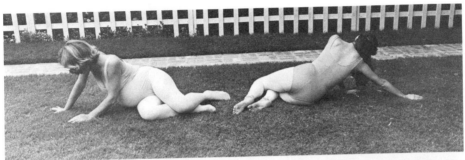

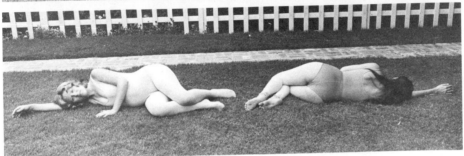

Pregnant Slide

Sit with your feet together, flat on the floor, knees bent. Let your legs fall to the floor on the right.

Place your left hand on the floor in front of your body, then slide your right arm back along the floor until you are lying on your side. Gently roll onto your back.

This exercise protects your abdominal muscles and allows you to lie down without strain or discomfort.

Many women complain that when they lie down they feel a strain on their abdominal muscles. When you learn to slide down on your side and then roll over on your back, you will avoid any sharp pains. You will also look and feel more graceful. You may not feel the need for this movement until your last three months, but you will be glad if you learn it early. You will be establishing a new pattern of motion.

Please don't lie straight back. I really scold the women who forget how to lie down the "pregnant way." It's so important to learn how to carry out this movement without straining your abdomen.

During labor this will be perhaps the only way you will be able to lie down. Cesarean mothers will also find this method to be essential for lying down during recovery.

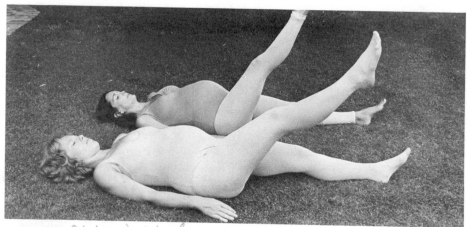

Leg Lifts *Abd + Waist, Legs*

Lie on your back. (Remember, do it the "pregnant way"!) Press your lower back gently into the floor. (Exhale as you lift one leg.) Straighten your knees as much as possible. Inhale as you lower your leg.

Repeat with your other leg, alternating sides as you continue.

When done properly, this exercise can stretch and strengthen your leg muscles while toning your abdominal muscles.

There is some question as to whether leg lifts are safe. Before attempting them, ask yourself these questions:
1. Are my abdominal muscles in good tone?
2. Was I exercising prior to my pregnancy?
3. Is my lower back pressed gently into the floor before I lift my leg?

If the answer to all three questions is yes, then you have no worry. If you answered the first two with a no, then I would suggest you modify the exercise. Lie on your back with one knee bent, your foot on the floor; then lift your other leg. Alternate sides, always keeping the passive leg bent.

A useful hint for doing leg lifts is to focus on imagery. Imagine you have tied a string around your foot. Now, attach that string to a pulley in the ceiling and let it lift your leg. As the string gets shorter, your leg lifts higher, with no strain.

Attitude can play a crucial part in all of these exercises. If you feel heavy, you will move accordingly. If you focus on images that help you feel light and graceful, your movements will flow. I danced and exercised right up until the day I delivered. So can you. You can create your own baby dance.

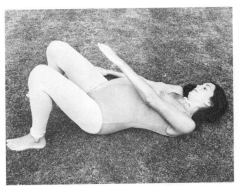 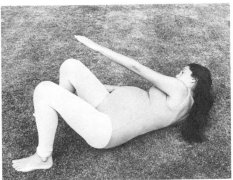

Tummy Toner *Abd & Waist*

Lie on your back with your feet flat on the floor, knees bent.

Tuck your pelvis under, pressing the small of your back on the floor.

Exhale as you reach with your right hand diagonally across your body, past the outside of your left knee. Lift your head and right shoulder off the ground.

Inhale as you roll your shoulder blades back onto the floor. Relax your neck and arm. Repeat on your other side.

Reaching across your body tones more than your abdominal muscles. You are toning the muscles that wrap around your torso as well. You are building a "girdle" to support your baby.

If you feel any tension in your neck when you lift your head and neck off the floor, let your head tilt toward the same side as the arm doing the reaching. Or, try putting your resting arm behind your head and lifting it. That way you can reach forward without tensing your neck.

One way to increase your endurance is to start by counting, "Reach up one, roll back one." Move with a smooth and even tempo. Be careful not to pop up too quickly. Progressively increase the count of each motion to five: "Reach up 2,3 4, 5, and roll back 4, 3, 2, 1." The slower you do this, the stronger your girdle will become. This exercise will help you to get back into shape more quickly by keeping your abdominal muscles in tone.

Make sure that you do not spend more than five minutes at a time on your back during your last trimester. If you feel light-headed or dizzy, roll over to your side, bending your knees. Breathe and relax.

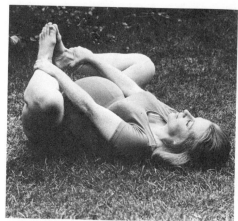 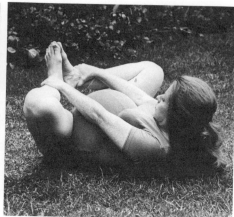

Alternate Tummy Toner *Abd + Waist*

Lie on your back, feet flat on the floor, knees bent. Bring the soles of your feet together, and let your legs open.

Hold onto your ankles, with your arms on the inside of your legs. Press your lower back into the floor.

Exhale and lift your head off the ground, looking between your feet. Inhale as you roll your shoulders and neck back onto the floor. Relax and repeat.

This exercise stretches your inner thighs while toning your abdominal muscles.

This exercise was useful for me when I was pushing my baby out. Opening my thighs and shortening my torso helped me bear down and push.

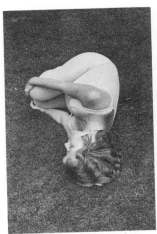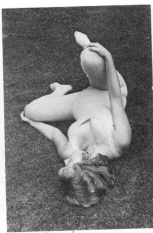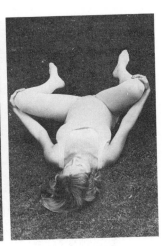

The Cradle _Buttocks, Back_

Lie on your back. Bring your knees toward your chest, holding onto your knees with your hands.

Gently rock to your side, letting your top leg close gently. Lift open your top leg far enough to create the need to roll to the other side.

Continue rolling from side to side. As you roll, let the momentum of your legs massage your lower back. This also stretches your inner thighs.

I always think of this exercise as a dessert. It feels so good. It is easy to do, too. Your baby is getting a great ride. And you've built your first cradle—organically.

Some women feel tender around their tailbones. If this exercise bothers you, put a pillow under your buttocks. Slow down the movement. If it is still painful, stop. You'll have a chance to enjoy the movement once your baby is born.

I couldn't get enough massage for my lower back when I was pregnant. This rolling was a welcome substitute.

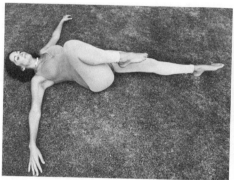 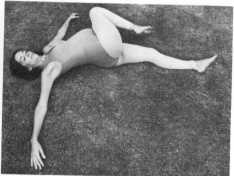

Lumbar Roll *Back, abd + Waist*

Lie on your back, legs outstretched. Slide your right foot up and bring your knee toward your chest.

Roll your leg across to your left side. Keep your right shoulder on the floor and twist your hip over until your right knee touches the ground.

Return the knee slowly, lowering your right hip back onto the floor. Slide your foot down. Repeat on the other side.

This exercise stretches your lower back and gives a gentle twist to your waist.

One of the best places to do this exercise is on a firm couch or bed. Let your top leg roll over the edge. You can stretch farther than if you were on the floor. If you don't have a firm couch or bed, the floor will do.

I found I needed to stretch my lower back daily. Sometimes I would hear a popping sound. My spine was adjusting, sending a rush of warm energy flowing through my lower back. Other times I simply enjoyed the stretch.

My baby seemed to favor my right side, leaving my back to compensate for the imbalance of weight. Lumbar rolls helped ease the strain. They can help your back too.

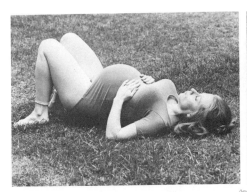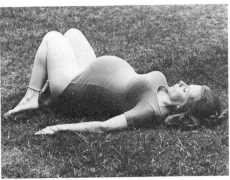

Tick Tock: A Pelvic Rocking Clock Back, Buttocks,

Lie on your back, feet flat on the floor, knees bent.

Inhale and press your lower back into the floor. Exhale and arch your lower back off the floor. Continue to alternate inhale/press and exhale/arch.

Next, imagine your pelvis as the face of a clock. Follow the second hand around, smoothly rotating your pelvis around in a circle. Press your buttocks and lower back into the floor as you rotate. Reverse direction.

Stop and lift your buttocks off the floor, raising your lower back up as you exhale. Inhale and slowly lower your spine onto the floor.

This series strengthens your pelvic girdle, lower back, and abdominal and upper leg muscles.

I found that this group of exercises let me feel as if I were dancing on the floor. I enjoyed the rhythms I could create by using different motions. I'm sure you'll enjoy this series, too.

Again remember, don't lie on your back too long during your last trimester.

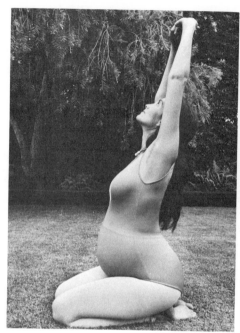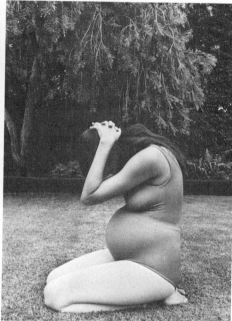

Mountain Pose *Ankles, Legs, Buttocks, Abd & Waist, Back*

Sit on your heels with your back straight.

Clasp your fingers and press your palms up, arching your back as you inhale. Look up and stretch your chin.

Exhale as you bring your hands down and rest them on the back of your head. Let your elbows relax and curl forward, chin to your chest.

Tuck your pelvis and lift off your heels. Sit back and down on your heels.

Repeat the cycle.

This exercise strengthens three sets of muscles: those in your thighs, abdomen, and lower back. It also helps to stretch your upper back muscles.

When you clasp your hands behind your head, let gravity work for you. Relax your elbows. Let them hang. Allow your neck and upper back to stretch from the weight of your arms and head.

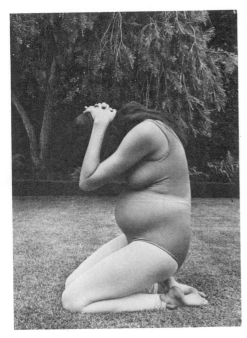

The crucial part of this exercise is making sure you have tucked your pelvis before you lift off your heels. Many women lean forward and don't feel the toning in their thighs. If you don't feel your thigh muscles, you aren't tucking your pelvis. Start over. Tuck your buttocks under. Now lift off your heels. This time, did you feel the pull in your thigh muscles? If so, you are on your way to beneficial "climbing."

When I first started to do this exercise I was amazed at how strenuous it felt. After a few weeks of practice, I felt fine. During my fifth month I had an opportunity to see if it really helped. I climbed a mountain with a friend. We went from 5,000 to 7,000 feet in a relatively short distance. My legs held up fine. It was my lungs that were challenged. I took it at a snail's pace, resting when I needed to, and made it to the top. We enjoyed the view, rested, and climbed back down. I'm not suggesting that you climb a mountain. But if there is a strenuous activity you enjoy, don't let your pregnancy stop you. Simply modify the pace to suit your needs.

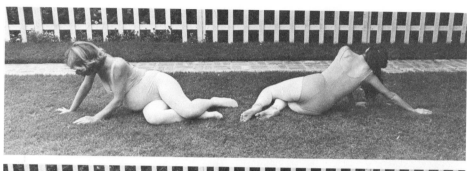

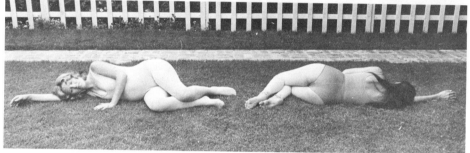

Getting Up

Lie on your back, arms at your side. Stretch your right arm and slide it up along the floor until it is next to your head, resting on the floor.

Bend your knees, sliding your feet along the floor. Let your legs lower gently to the floor on your right.

Bring your left arm across your body and roll toward your right side. Push down into the floor with your left hand, elbow bent. Slide your right arm toward your body as you sit up slowly.

To protect your abdominal muscles, getting up correctly is as important as proper lying down. This movement comes in handy for women who have to get up frequently in the middle of the night. The time may come when you can barely get out of bed. You'll be glad you know how to roll out, rather than trying to lift up and out like a turtle stranded on its back.

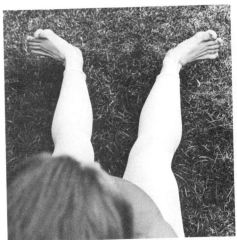 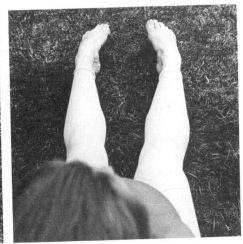

Ankle Works *Abd & Waist, Ankles*

Sit on the floor with your legs outstretched. Draw big circles with your toes, in both directions.

Take one leg and cross it over the other. Make a "comma" with your foot, swinging it back and forth, forth and back, as though you are keeping time to your favorite song. Repeat the movement with your other foot.

These easy circles and commas recirculate fluid back into your system, and can lessen swelling. They also strengthen your ankles and lower legs.

One of the benefits of this exercise is that you can build your ankles and legs without bearing the weight of standing up.

You can do these movements anywhere. I suggest to my students that they keep time with their favorite music, "conducting" with their feet.

Swollen ankles or sore feet may be telling you to relax more. Sit down and prop your feet up. Circle them and let the built-up fluid recirculate.

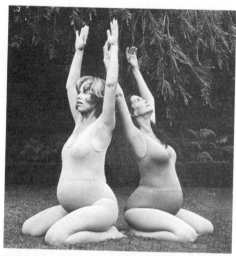

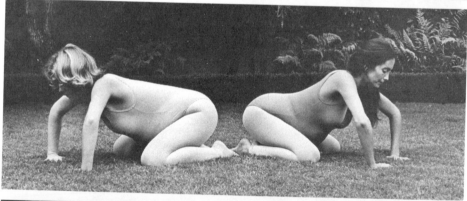

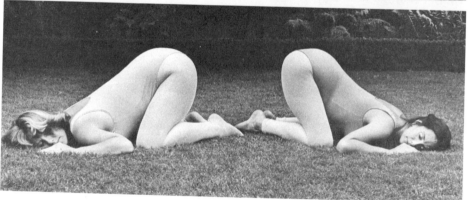

The Turtle Back

Sit on your heels, knees spread tummy-width apart.

Inhale and raise your hands over your head. Hiss as you exhale, lowering your hands to the ground, elbows bent. Lower your chest to the floor. Turn your head to the side and relax your arms.

Slide your hands around to your heels, then let your shoulders relax as you move them forward all the way to the floor.

Inhale, place your palms under your shoulders, and turn your forehead to the floor. Exhale and push up to your original sitting position.

This exercise stretches your lower back and helps to relieve gas. The discomfort of gas while you are pregnant demands immediate relief. This position is a blessing because it lets your baby fall forward, positions your bottom and gives the gas a passageway out.

As you grow larger, you may want to vary the position. Some women cross their arms in front, others put their bottoms higher in the air, still others spread their knees farther apart. Make whatever adjustment you need to feel comfortable.

I found this a great position for reading. It was one of the few times I was able to be on my stomach, or even close to it, while I was pregnant—especially during my last trimester.

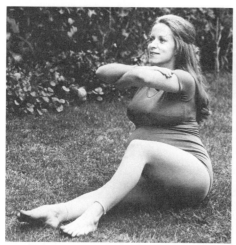 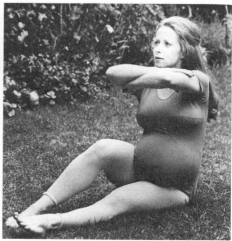

Buttocks Walk *Back , Buttocks*

Sit on the floor, legs stretched out straight in front of you. Fold your arms across your chest, elbows even with your shoulders.

"Walk" forward by lifting one hip up and sliding your leg forward, then lifting your other hip and sliding it forward.

Reverse and walk backward the same way. Repeat walking forward and back.

This exercise tones your buttocks muscles as you walk with them, and also strengthens your back muscles.

When we do this exercise in class, we form a circle and walk forward into the middle while singing a hearty tune. "The Caisson Song" (Over Hill, Over Dale) is a favorite. At the end of the stanza, we all stop and give a shout. This gives us a chance to tone our lungs while slimming our buttocks.

We rarely make noises except when we talk. However, when you are pushing your baby out, you may suddenly have an uncontrollable urge to grunt, or make a loud pushing sound. These sounds disturb some women; others find it a welcome release of tension. Practice loud and full sounds, or even a favorite song, with your coach. He will get used to you making loud sounds and won't be as startled if you do "roar" during your labor.

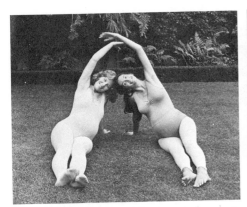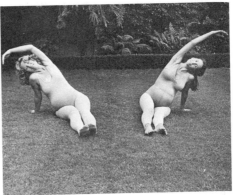

No Hips M'Lady *Abd & Waist, Legs*

Sit on the floor with your legs outstretched, your hands on the floor next to your hips.

Use one hand to push off and rock gently from side to side. As your hip leaves the ground the arm on the same side stretches overhead.

For a gentle twist for your waist, let your torso rotate toward the direction of the swing.

This exercise helps to break up fat tissue around your thighs and buttocks. Your arm motion also gives you a good stretch for your torso and waist.

Your baby creates many changes inside your body. One of the most visible is the weight gain in your hips and buttocks, most of which is necessary to help counterbalance the weight of the baby in the front. This extra flesh does not have to be flabby, though. You can be round and full and still be toned and firm.

I enjoyed the rocking and stretching. This exercise also helped me to breathe more easily. I had more space between my ribs and pelvis from the stretching. I couldn't help thinking my baby was enjoying the rocking too.

PARTNERING EXERCISES

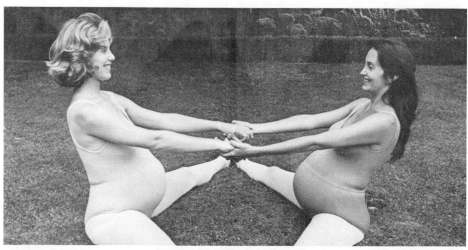

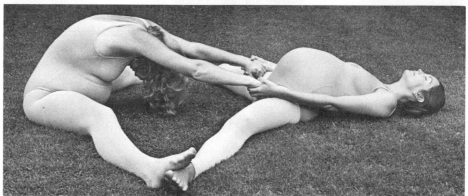

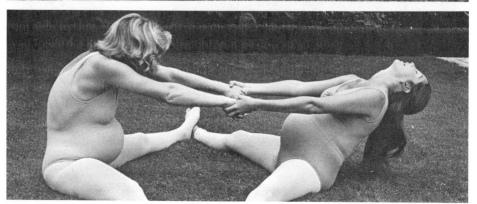

Partnering: Rowing the Boat Back, Abd & Waist, Legs

Sit on the floor facing your partner. Spread your legs apart with your partner's feet touching yours. Hold hands and rock gently back and forth.

As you rock back, inhale. Allow your chin to drop onto your chest, let your spine lower gently onto the floor, vertebra by vertebra, as far as you can go.

As your partner pulls you forward, exhale, using your lower back muscles to help lift you. Let your head drop back and relax your shoulders.

This exercise stretches your inner thighs and gently relaxes your legs at the hip joint.

The benefit of doing this with another person is that it helps both of you stretch. It also helps you to build trust in your partner to lower you slowly and safely. When you are lowering your spine to the floor, pull away from your partner to give some resistance. Gently roll your spine to the floor. If you lower straight back, without help, you might put too much strain on your abdominal muscles and possibly herniate them.

Curl your spine, don't drop it. Be gentle, please, no abrupt movements here. If either you or your partner are tight, let your knees bend as you reach forward. This allows a wider range of movement. It isn't important to lower your back all the way down to the floor at first. Rock gently back and forth and eventually your hips and thighs will stretch enough to allow you to relax your back all the way to the floor. I like to sing "Row, Row, Row Your Boat," but any song will do.

When you are pushing your baby out, you will need to know how to isolate your leg muscles and relax them. Leaving your legs open and relaxed while bearing down is an important skill. This exercise will help you acquire it.

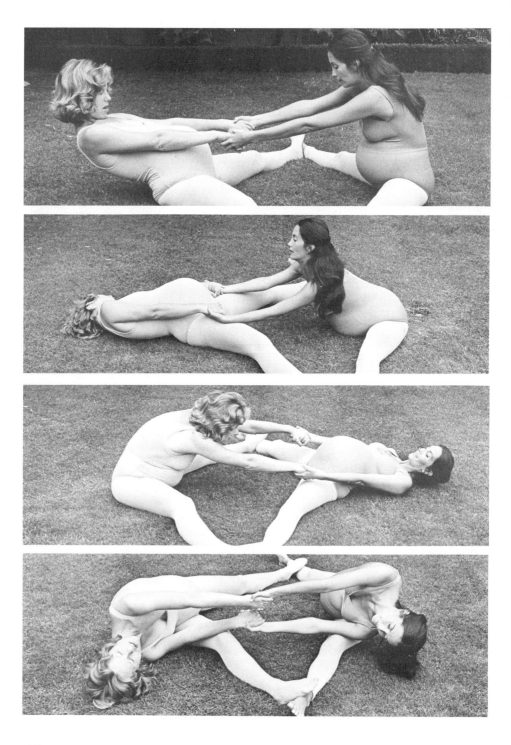

Partnering: Roll 'Em, Round 'Em Back, Abd & Waist, Legs

Sit on the floor facing your partner. Spread your legs apart with your partner's feet touching yours. Hold hands and pull your partner around in a circle, rotating your torso from the lower back up. If you can, let your shoulders and back roll on the floor. Breathe easily. Let your buttocks feel glued to the floor.

Reverse the direction of your circles.

This variation helps your lower back and hip joints with gentle circular motion.

Again, remember to keep a small amount of tension, pulling away from your partner. Allow your movement to flow smoothly. Roll one shoulder on the floor (or as low as you can), brush the floor with your back, then touch down with the other shoulder. Continue the circle, lowering your partner's shoulders. I love seeing the couples practicing this in a class.

Circles open a full range of movement in your hip joints. They help you to open your legs wide. You never know how long your second stage of labor will last; you may push for fifteen minutes, or as long as two and a half hours for your first baby. You want to build your endurance now, not during labor.

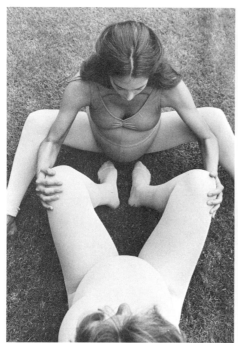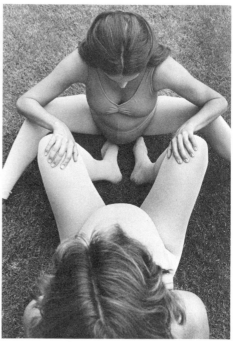

Kingdom Gates *Legs, Sh, Ch + Arms*

Partners sit on the floor facing each other. Beginning positions are as follows:

PARTNER 1: Place your feet together flat on the floor, knees bent. Put your hands on the floor behind your back and lean into your arms with your knees slightly apart.

PARTNER 2: With your legs spread apart, feet on the floor and knees bent, lean slightly forward and place your elbows on the inside of your knees with your hands on the outside of your partner's knees.

Partner 1 slowly spreads her knees apart as far as possible, while Partner 2 gives gentle resistance with her hands. When Partner 1's knees are as open as possible, both partners relax.

Partner 1 then slowly brings her knees together, with Partner 2 giving gentle resistance with her hands on the inside of her partner's knees. When Partner 1 has pressed her knees together, both partners relax.

Trade positions and repeat.

If two pregnant women are doing this exercise together, one partner is strengthening her arms and upper body while the other is stretching and isolating the muscles of her inner and outer thighs. The resistance should be strong, but not excessive. Don't clamp your partner's legs shut. Give firm, gentle pressure. Your legs need to work, not strain. Remember to breathe.

If you are Partner 2, when you press on your partner's knees, imagine you are sending a current of energy out your palms, through her knees to the floor. Be firm, not tense. Keep your elbows bent and your shoulders down. This can help you avoid putting tension in your neck and shoulders. After all, this isn't a contest to see who is stronger. You don't walk around on your hands all day.

This is another wonderful time to learn how to isolate your legs from your lower back. Many women will arch their backs as they push their legs open down to the floor. I remind them, and you, to relax your back and work on the muscles in your thighs. When you bring your legs together, you may experience trembling. This is good practice for those women who do experience trembling during transition in labor. Get used to the feeling and flow with the energy that creates the shaking.

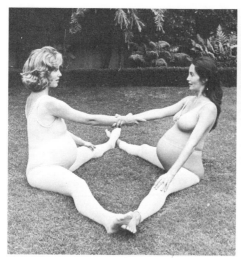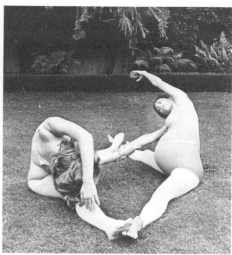

Partnering: Yea, Team *Abd + Waist, Legs*

Sit on the floor facing your partner. Spread your legs apart with your partner's feet touching yours. Shake hands and stretch your left arm over your head. Pull gently away from your partner.

Lean forward toward your right leg and exhale. Inhale as you lift up. Reach across and shake your partner's left hand.

Release your right hand, lift and stretch toward your left leg.

This exercise focuses on stretching and strengthening the muscles on the side of your torso, while stretching your inner thighs.

When you stretch up and then over, you increase the distance between your ribs and pelvic bones. Some women feel cramped in this area during pregnancy.

While you're pushing your baby out, you will need strong side muscles to help bear down. I can remember feeling short of breath during my ninth month. This exercise helped me to breathe and sit up more easily.

SAMPLE EXERCISE PATTERN

The following group of movements could serve as your basic daily exercise pattern. Supplement them with other exercises in this chapter according to your body's needs. Consult the Exercise Review Chart which follows for a breakdown of exercises by body part affected.

The Kegel Exercise
1. Tighten your vaginal muscles to a count of three as you inhale.
2. Exhale and relax the entire floor of your pelvis as you count to four.
3. 100 times daily.

Milkmaid
1. Standing with your feet parallel, tummy-width apart, take a cleansing breath (inhale through nose, hold, exhale through mouth).
2. Hold your arms straight out to the sides, palms facing forward. As you make 5 large circles to the sides, inhale with short sniffing breaths, for each circle.
3. Now make 5 circles in the opposite direction. Exhale with short sniffs, for each circle, as though you are blowing your nose.

Squatting Breath
1. Standing with your feet tummy-width apart, inhale, bringing your palms together over your head.
2. Lean forward, bending your hips, exhale as you bend your knees, coming down into a squat, lowering your arms in between your knees.
3. Keep your feet as parallel as possible. Do not roll in on your ankles and keep your heels on the ground if possible.
4. Inhale, straightening your legs. Bring your arms over your head as you return to a standing position.
5. Sigh as you let your arms float down to your side.
6. 3 times.

Head and Neck Rolls
1. Sitting with your legs crossed (Indian style), let your chin drop to your chest and roll your head slowly around, making a full circle.
2. Let your shoulders be relaxed. Sit tall and quietly.
3. Reverse direction.
4. 7 circles in each direction.

Pelvic Rocks
1. On your hands and knees.
2. Make sure your arms are directly below your shoulders and your legs are coming straight down from your hips, with space between your knees.
3. Tuck your pelvis under and forward, pulling up your abdominal muscles.
4. Now, let your tummy drop, and relax and sway your back into a gentle curve.
5. Continue the rocking action. Sway and tuck, sway and tuck. Be sure to isolate your lower back muscles, and avoid arching your upper back.
6. 20 rocks, 3 times a day.

Pregnant Slide
1. Use whenever you're lying down.
2. Sit with your feet together, flat on the floor, knees bent. Let your legs fall on the floor to the right.
3. Place your left hand on the floor in front of your body, then slide your right arm back along the floor until you are lying on your side. Gently roll onto your back.

Getting Up
1. Use whenever you're getting up.
2. Lie on your back, arms at your side. Stretch your right arm and slide it up along the floor until it is next to your head. Bend your knees, sliding your feet along the floor.
3. Let your legs fall gently to the floor on your right. Bring your left arm across your body and roll toward your right side. Push down into the floor with your left palm, elbow bent, and slide your right arm toward your body as you sit up slowly.

No Hips M'Lady
1. Sit on the floor with your legs outstretched, your hands on the floor next to your hips, elbows bent.
2. Use one hand to push off and rock gently from side to side.
3. As your hip leaves the ground the arm on the same side stretches overhead.
4. 20 rocks.

EXERCISE REVIEW CHART

Part of Body	Exercise
Head and Neck	— Head and Neck Rolls — The Wave: Soul Version and Open Version — Bucking Bronco — Wagging Your Tail
Shoulders, Chest, and Arms	— Single Arm Swings — Milkmaid — Thumbs Down — The Wave: Open Version — Kingdom Gates — Pelvic Rocks — Bucking Bronco — The Python
Wrists (all positions on all fours)	— Pelvic Rocks — The Python — Bucking Bronco — Wagging Your Tail

Back	— Head and Neck Rolls
	— The Wave: Soul Version and
	   Open Version
	— Supermarket Walk
	— Elevator
	— Squatting Breath
	— Monkey Walk
	— Partnering: Rowing the Boat and
	   Roll 'em Round 'em
	— Pelvic Rocks
	— The Python
	— Bucking Bronco
	— The Turtle
	— Mountain Pose
	— The Cradle
	— Lumbar Roll
	— Tick-Tock: A Pelvic Rocking Clock
	— Buttocks Walk
	— Raggedy Ann
	— Ankle Works

Abdomen and Waist	— Wagging Your Tail — Supermarket Walk — Lumbar Roll

105

Part of Body	*Exercise*
Abdomen and Waist (continued)	Partnering: Roll 'Em, Round 'Em and Yea, Team
	Tummy Toner
	The Wave: Soul Version and Open Version
	Partnering: All three versions
	Pelvic Rocks
	Mountain Pose
	Alternate Tummy Toner
	Raggedy Ann
	No Hips M'Lady
	Leg Lifts
Buttocks	Buttocks Walk
	Pelvic Rocks
	Tick-Tock: A Pelvic Rocking Clock
	Mountain Pose
	Bucking Bronco
	The Cradle
Pelvic Floor	Kegel Exercise
	Squatting Breath
Legs	Elevator
	Squatting Breath
	Monkey Walk
	The Wave: Soul Version and Open Version
	Partnering: All three versions
	Kingdom Gates
	Pelvic Rocks
	Bucking Bronco
	Mountain Pose
	Leg Lifts
	No Hips M'Lady
	Supermarket Walk
Ankles	Squatting Breath
	Monkey Walk
	Elevator
	Mountain Pose
	Ankle Works
Breathing	Abdominal
	Costal
	Candle-Blowing Breath
	Alternate Nostril

3. *Coaching: a labor of love*

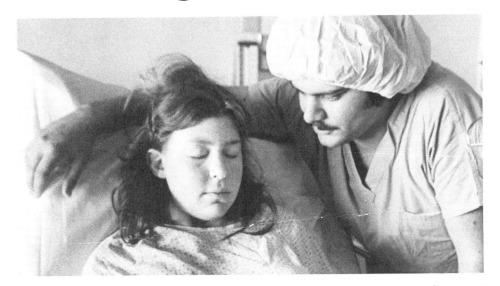

A labor of love, that's what your coach is offering you. While you are having the baby, he or she will be presenting you with a gift of love and support. So I am writing this chapter to the coach. It will be helpful for you to read it too, but it is dedicated to the person who is giving presence, not birth. For some women this person may not be the baby's father. For those of you who have chosen to share your birth experience with another woman or a male friend, please translate the pronouns into the appropriate one. Whoever the involved people are, be sure that they read this chapter.

THE IMPORTANCE OF COACHING

Coach or partner, you are a very important person. In order to make sensitive and educated decisions during the pregnancy, during labor, and after the baby is born, you will need training, too. You will need to know how to determine when there

107

are dangers and how to give comfort. If you and the future mother share your lives, you will be instrumental in creating a calm and relaxed atmosphere for the two of you. Coaching is a very creative process. There are definite skills and techniques you can learn, but as with any skill, it is the way you apply what you know that counts.

Let yourself explore the techniques and suggestions offered in this chapter. Don't feel compelled to "stick by the book." There are very few textbook pregnancies or labors. Each one is different.

Even if this is your first birth with your partner, you can approach it with faith in your ability to come up with creative solutions. Let your intellect and intuition work together. Trust yourself, but if you have any questions, don't hesitate to seek information. Most childbirth educators, nurses, and doctors are willing and able to help you—especially if you know how to ask.

In my classes I talk to my students about how to approach the health professionals to get information about pregnancy and birth procedures. Attitude is important. When you ask questions, show an openness and willingness to listen. Make it clear that you want their help, advice, or guidance. Approached properly, most people are happy to help you find the answers you need.

GETTING OFF TO A GOOD START

Your work begins long before labor. The "crisis" of birth usually has its origins in the months preceding delivery. How can you best offer support to the pregnant woman in your life? She isn't always the easiest person to live with. She tends to be fussy. She breaks into tears more easily. You're right when you sometimes think that the pregnancy is happening to both of you. You may even gain weight or experience morning sickness in true sympathetic form.

How closely do you want to connect with the pregnancy? Do you have any curiosity about what is happening inside the mother-to-be? Are you interested in seeing how the baby is developing? In Chapter 4 there is a section on fetal growth. If you would like to see more detailed color photographs, you might want to examine *From Conception to Birth* by Roberts Rugh and Landrum B. Shettles, M.D. It becomes easier to relate to the growth process if you can visualize what is happening within.

EXPLORING AND SHARING

For many couples in our society, the first baby may come at the same time as the man's push to establish his business or career. For some men this means an unexpected shift in plans. This needn't be a negative factor. Creative solutions exist if you are willing to search for them.

Take a good look at yourself. How do you feel about the baby? How will your life change once you become part of a family? How will the two of you get time alone? There are answers to all these questions. Explore them now with your partner, *before* the baby arrives.

What are *your* concerns? She doesn't have to be the entire focus just because she's pregnant. Share and communicate your needs with each other. It doesn't have to be one-way giving. Talk about your feelings, your fears, your joys. This is a time for closeness.

Discuss your childhood. Did you like the way your parents treated you? What did you swear you would never do to your own child? Parenting a first child is special. In some ways it is an experiment, a trial run. How do the two of you plan to approach it?

If you are having your second (or more), how will you share this experience with the other(s)? This is something to consider now. Sibling rivalry is real yet can be softened, especially when you take the time to share feelings and make special time for each member in your family.

Mutually agreeing on child-rearing philosophies and policies before the baby comes can help when parenting begins. It makes it possible to raise your child with a minimum of discord.

Perhaps you will want to learn more about pregnancy. There is literature written expressly for the expectant father. Reading it will help you know that you aren't the only one with mixed feelings.

SPENDING TIME TOGETHER

Pregnancy is a time of special intimacy. Remember, you will not have as much private time once the baby arrives.

As your pregnant partner's body changes shape and grows larger, it may become easier for you to relate to the reality of the baby. Many women don't really believe they will give birth until the baby starts to move. This is a time you can share. Put your hand on her tummy. Marvel with her at the movement. Here are some other pleasurable things you can do together:

Short-Order Fun

This is a fine time to get to know your kitchen. Flip through the cookbooks. Find recipes you can prepare. It's a delicious way to share time. She will need to eat better now that there are two to feed. *Better* is the key word here. Some of those cravings for sweets might really be a need for more protein. Your child's health will get a better start when Mom eats properly from whole, nutritious foods. Getting involved in the kitchen will prepare you for the time you might be needed as a short-order chef. During the first few weeks after delivery she may not feel like cooking.

Making Love

Some men love pregnant bodies. They enjoy seeing a woman round out with new voluptuous curves. Many women are radiant in a very special way during pregnancy.

Other men react differently. Yes, they still want to make love, but there is less urgency about it. Sometimes this hesitancy is due to a fear of hurting the baby. A lot depends on the woman. I discuss how she may feel in Chapter 1. If the water has broken, however, avoid penetration.

What it comes down to is that each couple need to discuss their own desires and preferences. What alternatives to penetration are there that might make you both feel pleasure? Is there something you would like her to do to you? And likewise, is there anything she especially likes that you could do for her?

Massage

For many couples, massage is a wonderful substitute for sex. Trade off—she gets one, then you (or whichever order feels right). You can also think of massage as a

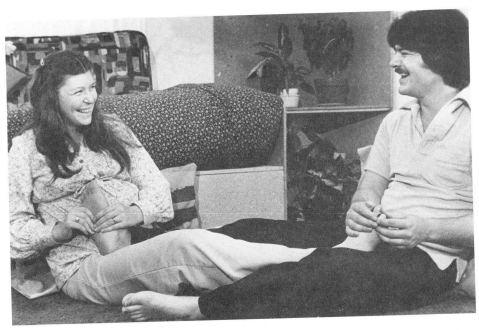

Massage helps you relax together

form of exercise. Massage stimulates blood and nerve circulation for the whole body. What a wonderful way to relax with each other.

Before you start, find a calm, private setting. It is important to have a quiet space with few distractions. Music is a wonderful way to enrich the atmosphere and add the right kind of accompaniment to your massage.

Different positions will feel more comfortable for a woman in different stages of pregnancy. In the last three months, lying flat on her back for long periods of time may bring on dizziness or light-headedness. The baby is pressing on the blood supply returning to the mother's heart, the *vena cava*. Instead, try a side-lying position or have her lean forward on pillows in a modified knee-chest position.

Remember to breathe when you are getting and giving a massage. We tend to forget to breathe when we are concentrating hard. Be aware of your entire body. Are you comfortable? If not, move or change your position.

What would feel good to you? Ask the person you are massaging what she enjoys. Many people are afraid to rub deeply, for fear it might hurt the other

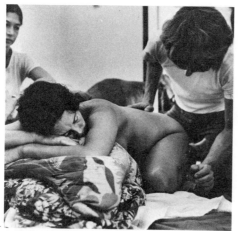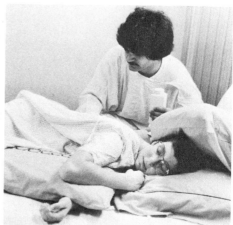

Massage can do wonders in easing labor

person. Don't be afraid to press right in and work out the tension or sore areas. Remember, feet are especially hardy.

If your mind wanders when you are giving a massage, refocus on what you are doing. Nothing is worse than getting a massage from someone who isn't there. The touch feels empty and often is not satisfying. Try to imagine that it is *your* body that is being rubbed. You will stay more connected to the massage.

Let yourself improvise; experiment with different combinations of techniques, strokes, types of oils, the music you play. Each massage can be different, exciting, and pleasurable.

Use the music to create a rhythm to rub to, or choose your own pace and flow with your breathing. Make sure the room is warm and comfortable or use blankets or towels to make things cozy.

Have some olive or other vegetable oil on hand. You may want to scent it or buy special oils. Oils rich in vitamin E (e.g., sesame, olive, almond, safflower) are wonderful food for the skin. Dimmed lights or candles can make a more intimate setting. Get into a comfortable position. Warm the oil in your hands. Music, maestro, please.

Massage Techniques

There are many different types of massage strokes. Find out which feels best for each of you. Movements include:

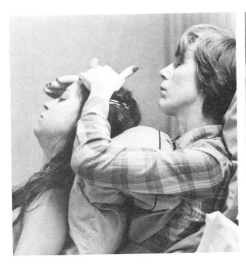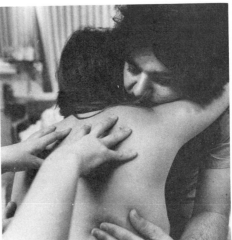

o A light stroke. Use the back of your hands to make long or short, circular or linear motions.

o Gentle fingertip action. Proceed delicately, barely touching, but be careful: some people are ticklish. Ask first.

o A light tapping motion. This can be very stimulating in a gentle way.

o Firm pressure. Press out tension with the palm or finger.

o Deep circular motion. Get into those tight places with the palm, thumb, or finger.

o Vibrating your palms or gently shaking with your hands.

o Cupping your hands and lightly clapping. This creates a vibration in the body that can loosen tension.

o Gently squeezing and releasing, as if kneading bread. This is especially effective for the neck and shoulder muscles.

o A tracing motion. Try spelling out pretend letters or making invisible designs or pictures.

Make sure your hands are warm before you start to rub. Icy fingers are a real shocker. Avoid sharp impacts or any direct blows to the spinal column. Work on either side of the spine. When massaging arms or legs, finish by stroking along the limb back toward the heart. This is a gentle way to promote circulation. A good way to relax a limb is to rotate it by holding the arm at the elbow, the leg at the knee. Start with small circles and enlarge them gradually. Maintain a slow, steady increase in tempo. This propeller-like motion releases tension in the joints. When you have finished circling the limb, straighten it out and pull it gently away from the body in a straight line. This helps to align the body.

We all seem to have chronic tension spots in our body. It is good to learn where your partner's are before labor begins.

Exercising Together

Exercising together is a pleasant and constructive way to share time. You might want to begin with stretching.

Stretching

Now lower your body to all fours and do *Pelvic Rocks* (see Chapter 2). This is an excellent lower back exercise for you, too. Let yourself have fun. Crawl around the room like playful animals.

Now, sit back to back. Put the soles of your feet together and do *The Wave* (see Chapter 2).

Back Talk

Start with your backs touching as much as possible. Let your chin lead out and pull your body forward in a smooth, rolling motion. When you bring your chin

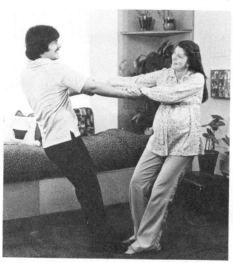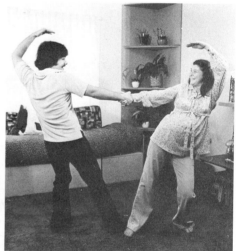

Stretching

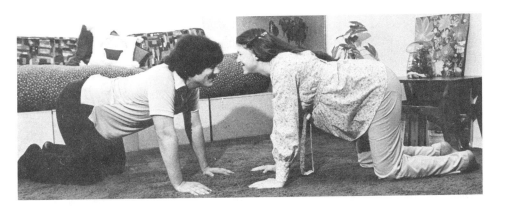

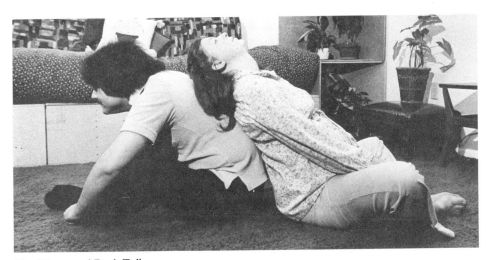

The Wave *and* Back Talk

back to your chest and start to roll your spine back up to a seated position, let your backs gradually roll together. Play with this exercise.

Let one person lead the movement and the other person follow. Sway and move as if you were Siamese twins joined at the spine. Allow your legs to move as is necessary to let you stretch and move as freely as possible.

Rowing the Boat
This is a good exercise for both of you. It stretches your inner thigh and lower back muscles. Try singing as you row. The tenderness you experience while

115

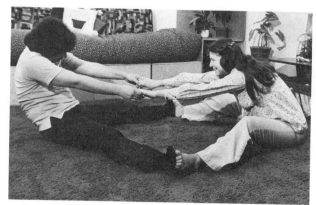
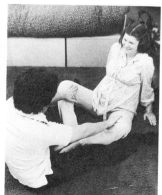

Rowing the Boat   Kingdom Gates

stretching your leg muscles is similar to what an early contraction will feel like. Try to breathe into the tight muscle. It is possible for you to have some sensation of what labor might feel like. Do all of the partnering exercises (see Chapter 2) and add sounds to them. Often singing, either one note or a whole song, or making breathing or hissing sounds, can involve more than one sense in the action. Use your whole being when you exercise. Think of images that will enhance the experience. When you are doing *The Wave*, think of the ocean. Visualize waves in your back.

When you are doing the partnering exercises, feel the atmosphere around you getting thick, as if it were filled with whipped cream or pudding. Move through it slowly, with light resistance. When you do the *Kingdom Gates* (Chapter 2), let your partner feel strong, too. Don't push down too hard or fast. After all, you walk on your legs, they had better be stronger than her arms!

Find other physical activities to do together. Some couples enjoy bicycling together. Others jog. I have seen women at the YMCA I belong to jogging into their ninth month. They run at a slower pace than most of the group, but that doesn't matter. Pregnant women can still use aerobic exercises to tone the cardiovascular system. You might benefit from the exercise, too.

Swimming is a wonderful way to spend time together. She will love it because it is one of the few times she can feel weightless. Take walks together after dinner. Go out dancing. Disco is a fine activity for pregnant women. Most of it is foot or arm work anyway. Her hips are still mobile. I got so many warm and encouraging remarks from people whenever I would go out dancing. People really love to see pregnant women in public.

EMOTIONS DURING PREGNANCY

For many couples, pregnancy is a time of change, even crisis. How does the woman explain fears to her partner when they seem unreasonable even to her? She will not be sleeping as much, and her wakefulness might disturb your sleep. One suggestion is, budget allowing, to get a bigger bed if yours is currently too small. You both need to sleep. She will be getting up to go to the bathroom, will move from restlessness, or will be awakened by the baby's movements. Just as you've drifted off to sleep again, you may be called upon to banish a nightmare. Pregnancy is notorious for dreams that can wake a woman up from a sound sleep and leave her feeling upset. Dreams about the baby's being hurt or something going wrong at birth are all common types of anxiety dreams that women have during pregnancy. I can remember a dream I had in which I gave birth to an owl and it was too small to nurse. By listening actively and supportively to her fears, you can be very reassuring. Try not to push aside her fears with "Oh, you're just dreaming. Go back to sleep." *Be there* for her.

At the same time, let her know your feelings. Don't blame her for them but let her know how her actions or your own fears are affecting you. She wants more hugs and you may want more space. Both of you have your needs. Do your best to find a healthy middle ground. You might each plan to spend a night alone, or with a friend. Plan to spend quality time with each other, not just those weary moments at the end of a long day.

PRACTICE MAKES PERFECT—A TIME DISTORTION TECHNIQUE

One coaching technique I have found extremely useful involves practice before the labor. You can start now if you wish. What you will be doing is bringing rest and pleasure into the labor by calling on places, times, and sensations that are relaxing

117

and pleasurable. Play around with these three basic elements. You may find more of your own. All you need is a watch with a second hand and a quiet place to lie down or sit together.

Have her close her eyes. Let her relax for a moment. Ask her to uncross her feet and/or hands. Now, you will gently (without tickling) talk to her and touch her body to reinforce the relaxation process. Start with her feet. Ask her to relax each foot as you touch them. Moving your hands up to touch her lower legs, knees, thighs, buttocks, entire back, abdomen, chest, shoulders, arms, hands, neck, face, and scalp.

This completes the relaxation phase. Next, tell her that she will have one minute of clock time to experience as much rest as she needs. When you dream, you can distort time to make a minute feel more like an hour, a day, or a week. This is a very similar process. Ask her to give herself permission to rest and relax as much as she needs. Tell her when the minute starts. Don't talk during that time. Be together quietly. When the minute is over, use a soft voice to tell her.

Ask her to slowly come back to the room and open her eyes. Reassure her that she will feel rested and relaxed when she does so. Find out what it was like for her. Share the experience. She can then try the same technique on you. It's a wonderful way to help each other relax.

A variation on this involves imagining pleasurable places or things you both enjoy. Begin by getting her relaxed and in touch with her body and breathing. Repeat the relaxation process. Then let her know that for one minute of clock time (or whatever length of time you wish) she will go to her favorite place or engage in a favorite activity. However, in her imagination she can stay there for as long as she needs. At the end of the clock time you will gently call her back to the room. Assure her that she will return feeling relaxed and refreshed. Have her get in touch with her breathing again, and ask her to open her eyes when she is ready.

Still another variation on the above deals directly with the process of labor and delivery. Repeat the relaxation phase, then have her "see" or experience her labor in the most positive fashion for one minute of clock time. Ask her to visualize the baby being born and see herself holding it in her arms. Complete the process as before. This is a very powerful experience for many women. Others find such visualization more difficult, but with practice they can use it to help create a positive labor experience.

Putting Practice to Work When It Counts

How can I use these visualization techniques during labor, you may ask? How will they help? These are good questions. The answer is that they can be utilized any time during the first stage of labor. They are especially useful when there are at least two minutes between contractions and she is feeling tired or her energy is low.

The first time I put one of these techniques to the test as a coach in a labor situation, the woman had never done the exercises before. Her labor had started out with contractions three minutes apart, fast and heavy, but when she got to the hospital her contractions got weaker. Unfortunately, she didn't feel them as weaker; she was still remembering how the earlier ones had felt. Her husband had come down the hall to get me and he seemed upset. She was very tense during the contractions, clearly not "on top" of them. Her Peruvian ancestry came out when she started to cry, "Aye, Aye." I encouraged her to use the sound, but not to get tense doing so. Sound can be a powerful tool in labor—singing, moaning, groaning, growling—whatever comes naturally. "Elysa, I'm so tired, I just can't go on," she insisted. "Okay, let your husband have the baby and let's leave," I replied. She looked at me incredulously and then started to laugh. That moment of humor got us past her resistance, and she returned to accepting the process and was able to go on. What she wanted to do most was to rest. So, we used the time-distortion technique. I had her go "in" for one minute of clock time and rest "for as long as she needed to." She came out of that minute with her face looking more relaxed and her whole body more prepared for the next contraction, which started one half minute after she opened her eyes. We did it again after the next contraction; this time she "went shopping." When she opened her eyes there was a big grin on her face. Her husband asked her what had happened. She explained that she had bought a new dress.

This couple was able to use this technique during the rest of the labor; it gave them something constructive and pleasurable to do. He was able to help his wife rest, relax, and experience a moment's break in the laboring period.

CHILDBIRTH CLASSES

Toward the end of the pregnancy, one night a week might be spent going to a childbirth preparation class. More and more doctors are recommending them and for most couples it is the most exciting part of the pregnancy. There are several methods for you to choose from: Bradley, Harris, or Lamaze. They all present information about labor and delivery, its emotional and physical stages, hospital procedure, and possible complications, and also give you valuable postpartum preparation. Breathing skills and relaxation methods are stressed. Questions about how to prepare for birth are answered.

The classes can last for five to ten weeks. I suggest you sign up early to make sure that you get the class you want and to ensure that you are able to finish the course before the baby is born. Occasionally babies do come earlier than scheduled. You can start during the sixth or seventh month.

These classes also offer you a chance to meet other expectant fathers. Find a father who has attended his child's birth. Ask him about it. It may help prepare you for your own experience. Hopefully your instructor will encourage talk and sharing of feelings among the men in the class.

DANGER SIGNS DURING PREGNANCY

An important part of your duty as coach is to keep alert for signs of possible trouble. In the unlikely event that any of the following happens, call your doctor at once.

○ profuse vaginal bleeding
○ a sudden puffiness or swelling around the joints that restricts movement
○ dizziness
○ a weight gain of over ten pounds in one week (hers, not yours)
○ any abnormal swelling in the abdomen that could indicate internal bleeding

LABOR—TRUE OR FALSE?

As the big day draws near, you will begin to wonder how you will know when labor really begins. We've all heard stories of taxicab deliveries but it rarely happens that quickly for the first one. Usually from the time a woman first recognizes that she is in labor, there are three to thirty hours more until the baby is actually born. The signs of true labor beginning are:

○ change of mood to calmness or serenity
○ breaking or leaking of the water sac, which is filled with amniotic fluid. This is a clear liquid. If you see fluid that is dark or muddy-colored, call the doctor.
○ passing of a bloody show. That happens when the mucous plug dislodges from the mouth of the uterus (cervix) as it effaces, gets thinner, and then begins to stretch open and dilate.

○ irregular cramps or intermittent backaches which become more and more regular, lasting longer than 45 seconds, and 3 to 5 minutes apart
○ A sudden urge to remodel the living room.

Not all women experience a calmness, but it is a pleasure to be around those who do. They just "know" that the baby will be born soon. Don't try to find out why or how she knows. Most will just say, "I have a feeling, that's all."

Make sure you have everything ready for the birth, your hospital bag or any other equipment you will need, *at least two weeks before* the baby is scheduled. Don't be one of those who arrive at the hospital totally unequipped because labor came sooner than anyone expected. Be prepared—just like the Scouts! You are the counselor here. See that the camper is packed and ready to go.

Occasionally labor will start and stop. As long as the water bag hasn't broken, this is nothing to be concerned about. I remember one lady calling me up for a week running in the middle of the night before her daughter was born to ask me if she was really in labor. Each time, her "cramps" would fizzle out. I suggest that if this happens to your partner and you aren't sure if she is really in labor, you have her get up and go for a short walk around the house. If the contractions stop, labor was just staging a dress rehearsal. If, however, labor picks up and gets stronger, chances are this is the real thing.

COACHING DURING LABOR

Stage One

Most first labors start slowly. First the cervix thins out. Then it will start to stretch or dilate to a full 10 centimeters (4 inches) in diameter. The first stage of labor is complete when the cervix has stretched open completely. That process can take from three hours, in a fast labor, to 28 hours for first babies. For the second and subsequent babies, it could be as short as one to five hours, so be prepared for anything with second children. But here again, remember that each labor and delivery is different. Be prepared to observe and improvise.

I remember one friend who kept denying she was in labor. "No, Elysa, those are just gas pains." When we timed the pains they turned out to be suspiciously regular. She wanted to wait until her doctor came back on duty (which wasn't until the following morning) before she had the baby. She kept asking me to go home; I knew better. Her husband wasn't due home until six, and I didn't want

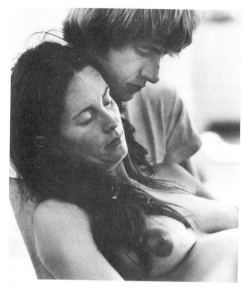

Help her with her breathing

to leave her alone in labor. She took naps and rested; I gave her back rubs and massaged her feet. She did most of the work for the first six hours. She breathed, relaxed, and responded well to any suggestions to relax her shoulders or other tight body parts.

For other women, myself included, labor started with a bang, not a whimper. My contractions started three minutes apart and lasted for 45 to 60 seconds. I was amazed, however, at how little actual pain there was at this stage. Slow, relaxed breathing and a bit of encouragement from my friends were sufficient during the early phase of labor.

Once labor starts, make sure she doesn't eat anything heavy. Her stomach won't be able to digest food. Give her tea, juices, or perhaps a clear broth. If she does eat, she will probably vomit it up later during labor. This is normal but best avoided.

Many of the couples I have taught said they liked to cuddle during the beginning of labor. They find this a wonderful time to be close. After all, it is this kind of energy that made the baby, so why not let it ease the infant out into the world. She can walk around, if she likes. Let her do a little fussing here and there,

122

but don't let her overdo it. Her energy is needed for the labor, not housecleaning or major projects. If you need help, call on your friends.

Help her to begin her labor relaxed by aiding her with her breathing. This will establish a solid foundation for the rest of the labor. If you can, lie in bed and have her sit up in between your legs, with her back against your stomach. Put your hands on her belly and feel what the first contractions are like. Breathe with her. Gently remind her to breathe fully and relaxed. This is nice to do as a warm-up, even before labor starts or as a practice technique. You could also rub her belly in that position, making slow circles with a light and gentle touch. It's called effleurage. You might want to use powder or cornstarch to help your hand glide more easily.

For many women, this stage is fairly easy to "ride." Your partner might even be talking to you during a contraction. I have often talked to women on the phone while they were in labor, and they will start to breathe more deeply and excuse themselves, saying, "Here comes another one, just a moment." As the coach, you will know when labor gets heavier. She won't be talking as much, she will want you to stay closer. Remember, you are a source of reassurance and strength to her.

The beginning contractions, during which time the cervix is opening to 4 centimeters, often are 5 to 20 minutes apart and last for 30 to 60 seconds. Before labor gets heavy, you could be the one to help her with an enema. That way you can clear out the lower passages in the rectum. Enemas tend to speed up labor in a gentle way and are certainly more pleasant early in labor than later on. Make sure when you give her an enema that she is in a knee-chest position, or the water won't go in. The baby's head will prevent it unless her buttocks are raised and the shoulder lowered. This should be discussed with the doctor, who should be told what your plans are before you go to the hospital. A warm bath can also feel wonderful, *if* the waters haven't broken. Once the waters break, showers are suggested to make sure no foreign matter is floated into the uterus. Each doctor has his or her own policy regarding when you should go to the hospital. In most cases, they want you to leave home when contractions have stabilized at around three minutes apart and are lasting 45 to 60 seconds. This is a sign that the woman is entering the active phase of labor. You will need to remind her to urinate every hour or so. *This is critically important.* The bladder is very small now and it is to her advantage to make sure it stays empty.

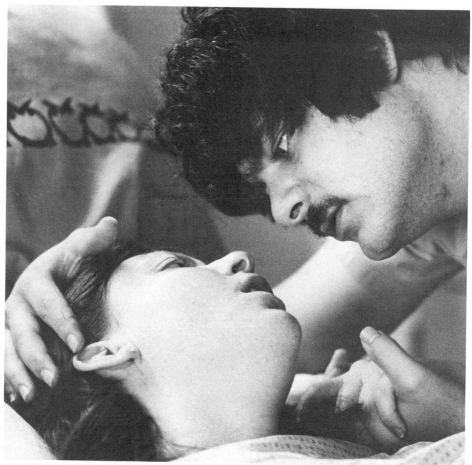

During this phase, the coach plays a more active role

The Active Phase of Labor

During the active phase, in which the cervix will dilate to 7 or 8 centimeters, you will play a more involved role. She will need to concentrate more with each contraction. You can use your voice to help soothe her. I enjoyed hearing my coach talk about rivers and streams running through my body to let all the tensions out. The more you flow with the labor, the more smoothly it will progress. Tenseness can slow things up. Don't demand too much of her or yourself, however. There are some things neither of you can control.

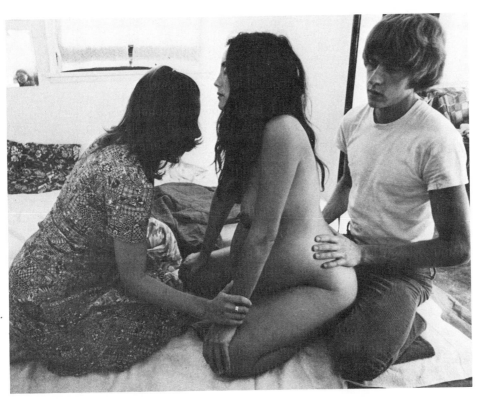

Counterpressure in the lower back can help

As the active phase progresses, you might want to give counterpressure in the lower back. This is where the massage techniques you practiced will count. Some teachers suggest rolling tennis balls or using rolling pins on the back. This can help you; coaches get tired, too. You might want to have a back-up. Many hospitals allow two people into the labor room. If you have a back-up you can leave and rest for a while.

Time Out for the Coach

To find an alternate, think about some of your fellow students in the childbirth classes. You might know another person who is pregnant or who has recently had a child. These women make wonderful coaches. Abbey, who was one of my coaches, was tremendously helpful. I had been at her son's birth three months before—the first birth I had ever seen. She was perfect at my labor. She massaged my back and feet, sat behind me, whispered in my ear, stroked my brow with a cool washcloth, and gave my coach a needed rest.

Pick-up Exercises for the Coach

Here are some exercises for you to do to unwind and get your circulation going. These are simple and can be done during labor. Think of it as your half-time break.
1. Shake your body all over, and move as many parts as you can. If you are having trouble finding a quiet space, ask the nurse if there is a doctor's sleeping room available for you to use for a short time. If not, the father's waiting room often has a bathroom attached and you can use that.
2. Put your hands on your shoulders and circle your elbows, both going the same direction; then reverse the direction. Now try each arm going in a different direction (not quite like patting your head and rubbing your stomach, but close).
3. Let your head flop forward and do easy *Head and Neck Rolls* (see Chapter 2); breathe in as you circle your head back, and exhale as your head rolls forward. Let it relax any neck tensions you have stored.
4. Circle your hips. Put your hands on your lower back, and circle one direction, then the other.
5. Stretch your legs, in almost any fashion that you can. Stretch your calves, bring

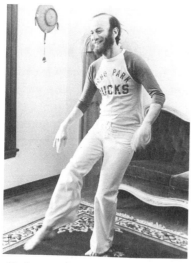
Shake your body

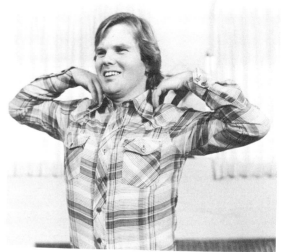
Elbow circles

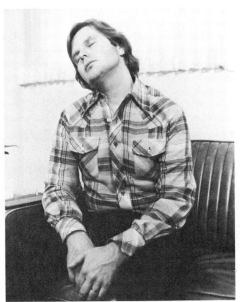

Head and Neck Rolls

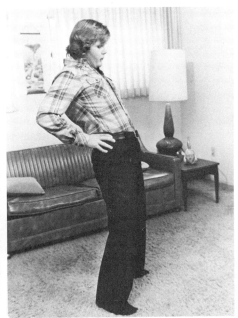

Hip circles

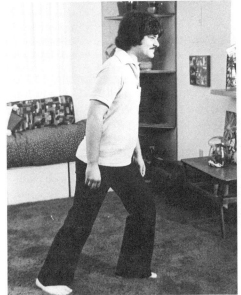

Stretch your calves

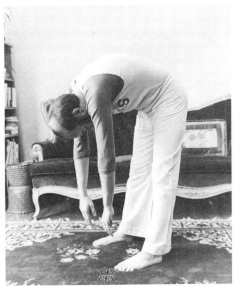

Bend over

your knee toward your chest to stretch out your lower spine, swing your leg, bend forward and try to touch your toes. Let the circulation return to your legs. When you bend over, it will also flush out your head a bit. Feel the blood going into your brain and refreshing your capacity to be clear-minded.

6. Give your body gentle cupping slaps all over, as described in the massage techniques section. That can refresh your system in a jiffy. Pat your arms, legs, stomach, as much of your back as you can reach, and your face and head.

7. If you are really feeling adventurous, run up and down a few flights of stairs. That will give you a quick lift and get you breathing more fully.

8. Sit down and relax. You might want to eat a small amount, if it has been a long labor. Let your back-up take over while you rest.

9. Be aware of your breathing. You might want to imagine you are in your favorite place for a short while. You deserve to feel some pleasure today, too.

The Importance of Relaxation

Note your partner's language during the active phase of labor; it will telegraph a lot about how she is handling the contractions. Labor is one of those unique processes that you are best off letting happen. The woman needs to surrender to the process as much as possible and let her body dilate and stretch. I think that is the hardest part of the first stage of labor. You can't really do anything but relax, breathe, and let the body open up to be able to push the baby out.

If you see any part of her body tense, help her relax it. Use your hands or your voice to gently remind her to let go. Remember, you are her guide. If she is uncomfortable in one position, suggest another one. Look at the birth pictures in Chapter 5 to get ideas. Looking into her eyes can help her establish contact with this world. There is a tendency for some women to want to fade away when the contractions start feeling strong. Their eyes roll back in their head, or they move in a manner that is fighting the contraction, not moving with it. The intensity of the stretching is amazing. I remember that I was constantly astounded that my body could experience and tolerate so much and still come back to a feeling of relaxation in between contractions. Coaches helped tremendously by reminding me to relax and breathe. They reminded me of what was happening: "Elysa, you are stretching, not injured—let your cervix open."

Transition

The stage in which the cervix is coming into the home stretch—8 to 10 centimeters—probably has the worst reputation of any stage of labor. It comes right before the second stage, in which the woman will start to feel the urge to push. This is a time for you to stand by. Fortunately, it tends to be a short part of the whole process. Transition can last from 15 minutes to 2 hours. You are very definitely needed *now*.

Some of the signs of transition are:

o A bloody show.
o The urge to push.
o Belching or passing gas.
o Nausea. If the vomit looks bright green, don't be alarmed; it is usually caused by the liver secreting more bile into the system.
o Greater rectal pressure; she might say she wants to have a bowel movement. That is the head moving further into the birth canal.
o A sudden mood change.
o Possible trembling all over her body, or in the legs. This is normal and indicates a surge of adrenaline and energy going through the body to help stretch the cervix the final 2 or 3 centimeters. Remember when you practiced the *Kingdom Gates* together? The trembling you might have experienced bringing your legs together is very much like what she is experiencing now. You can help by coaching her breathing. Keep it slow and steady. She needs more oxygen now, but panting can create hyperventilation and tire her out needlessly.

The hardest part about transition is that the contractions are longer and more frequent. They may last for 60 to 90 seconds, with only a minute in between. Therefore it is hard to find time to relax. Help her in any way you can. Massage her, blow on her face, rub her back, listen to her breathing and breathe with her, talk to her and remind her that this is the home stretch. Soon she will be able to push the baby out. In between contractions, remind her of any pleasant or pleasurable sensations.

She is apt to say strange things. There is very little blood in her head. Be patient, kind, and loving. Don't take anything personally that she says to you now, unless it is positive, of course. One woman turned to her coach during the peak of her transition and asked him if he had eaten. She was showing concern for him.

Women can also be kind during transition. Ina May Gaskin in *Spiritual Midwifery* talks about the importance of giving to the man during labor.

Try to talk about what both of your fears about transition are and figure out what techniques might help. You might have to change them entirely during labor, but you will at least have had time for dress rehearsals.

Stage Two: Pushing

I went to sleep during transition. Amazingly I found myself getting drowsier and fading off. My contractions got less intense and I napped for 45 minutes. This was my body's way of rejuvenating for the big push.

Once labor was under way, I had strong contractions. It felt like one came almost right after the other. I felt like pushing before I was really ready. When that happened, my coach helped me to blow slowly, but *not* to go with the urge to push until I was fully dilated. The panting and blowing worked as a distraction, helping me relax and breathe through contractions without pushing.

How do you, as a coach, know when she's ready to push? Another good question. A nurse or the doctor will do a vaginal exam to check that she is in fact fully dilated.

When she *does* become fully dilated, you can help her push this new bundle of life out into the world. Try to get behind her, or prop her up with pillows. She can't push as easily when she is lying flat on her back. Perhaps she will push more effectively if she lies on her side. Some women do. In that case, lift her top leg and hold it while giving her explicit coaching instructions.

Instructions to the Coach for Pushing

1. Have her inhale gently, exhale, inhale. Ask her to drop her chin to her chest and hold her breath.
2. When she bears down, that is, pushes (holding her breath for the whole countdown), count down rapidly from 10 to 1, interjecting encouragement every now and then. "Ten, nine, eight, good, six, five, that's fine, three, two, almost there, now exhale slowly." Have her exhale with her mouth open fully and slowly to maintain the baby's progress out of the uterus (you will want her to push three times during each contraction).
3. A full cycle of a push consists of this: First have her inhale lightly—flutter the breath in with short inhalations (or sniffs); she should not suck in the air forcefully; that only encourages tension in the upper chest and can reverse the progress

made bearing down. After inhaling in this way, she drops her chin to her chest, holds and pushes (while you count down), then exhales. Slowly she inhales gently again. She holds, drops the chin to the chest, you count down, she pushes, exhales, and relaxes. The contraction is probably over.

If the contraction is over before you complete a full cycle (three pushes), don't worry; you will get another try. I have seen first babies come out in four pushing contractions. I personally took two hours to push my daughter out. I was amazed at how long it took me to learn how to push effectively. You will often hear it likened to pushing out a constipated stool. It is somewhat like that, except you relax and push at the same time. It seems like a contradiction—pushing and relaxing—but it is possible. I kept visualizing flowers blooming, golden lotus blossoms with a thousand petals, each opening one at a time. Once the head started to come out, I experienced a stinging around the lips of my vagina. My breathing helped, but it was definitely my concentration that was needed. My coach reminded me to relax, especially my jaws. Somehow I thought, "If I clench my jaw, the baby will come out easier." Wrong. In fact, there is a curious correlation between having your jaw and throat relaxed and open and enabling the pelvic floor and vagina to stretch more easily.

One thing to remember about pushing is that when the head starts to come out, encourage her *not to push.* Let her "breathe" the head out. If she pushes too hard, she can tear. Doctors generally give episiotomies, an incision in the perineum, to make the vagina a bit larger. If your doctor is open to alternatives, you might suggest that you give her a gentle perineal massage with a lubricant during labor. My coach used olive oil to rub my perineum. Right before the head started to descend, he also applied hot compresses to the area—folded Kotex dipped in water. The slowness of my daughter's descent, plus the massage and the hot compresses, made it unnecessary for me to have an episiotomy. Many women could avoid an unnecessary incision if given this care. Episiotomies must, like any other kind of wound, heal. I have seen twelve-pound babies delivered vaginally without an episiotomy. The doctor is the critical part of the team here. Talk with him beforehand and ask him if he would be willing to help you try to avoid this procedure. Some doctors are very willing to try. For others this may be a new request. Remember, tearing can be avoided by taking a few preliminary precautions. To repeat: massage the perineum and use hot compresses. Have her breathe the baby's head out, not push. Put gentle counterpressure on the perineum. That way the head won't rush out so quickly.

The two of you did it. The baby is here.

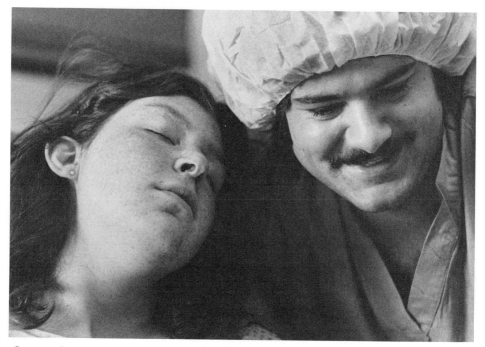

Congratulations, coach; congratulations, Mom

For some men, having a son first is very important. One father I remember rather unfondly looked at his beautiful newborn daughter and lamented, "Too bad, dear, it's a girl, better luck next time." What an insensitive welcome into this world. Look at your desires before the birth. Discuss your reactions to a boy or a girl. How would either sex affect your ability to relate to that child?

Third stage, expulsion of the placenta, is crucial for the mother's health, because once the baby is born the placenta separates from the lining of the uterus and becomes a foreign body. Generally within half an hour after the baby is born the uterus contracts and expels the placenta. Stimulation, sucking or pulling, on the nipples helps the uterus contract, if there is any problem.

ABDOMINAL BIRTH: CESAREAN MOMS

If your partner is offered medication during labor, find out if it is really necessary for the health of the baby. If you are told it is, cooperate. If it is being offered for the mother alone, this becomes a personal decision. There are really no "safe drugs" in childbirth. They all have an effect on the mother and the baby. When they are given later in labor, there is less time for the drugs to have an influence. There is often less *reason* to give drugs then, too. This is where the coach is invaluable.

The mother's job is to preserve and promote her health and the health of the baby. Whatever is best for both is what she will want to do. The most common reasons for this procedure are:

o The head is too large to fit through the pelvis.

o The cervix is not dilating even with pitocin—often called failure to progress.

o There is some indication that the baby is in distress and must come out immediately.

o There is some indication that the mother is in distress and the baby should come out immediately.

o The baby is in a breech or an unusual position (first child), which means the feet (or buttocks) are down in the canal (picture the baby standing up instead of head down).

There are a surprising number of Cesarean births today. The national average is between 15 and 25 percent, and in some hospitals it's over 40 percent. Given the figures, it is important that you discuss beforehand how you would feel if you needed an emergency Cesarean. In some hospitals the husband is allowed to come into the operating room; in others he is asked to wait in the father's waiting room. Find out what the policies are at the hospital you've chosen. If you are included in the operating room, you will be asked to get into a scrub suit and stand by her shoulders. Many anesthesiologists do not use a general anesthesia, but give epidurals or spinals so that the woman is wide awake for the operation and the birth. She can see the baby and will be able to talk to you, but feels nothing from the waist down. For those women who do have a general anesthetic, ask the doctor if you can hold the baby after it is born. Many doctors are very helpful in promoting the bonding process for families.

Bonding is being talked about more and more lately. It is the process of connecting with the baby once it is born. They can see, providing the light isn't too bright or the drops haven't been put in their eyes right away. There is a special closeness men and women feel at the completion of the birth. The child is here and you want to see it, touch it, count the fingers and toes. All the joy of nine months of waiting is there to be shared with your newborn.

THE INCREDIBLE JOURNEY

One last issue must be dealt with so you will be fully prepared for childbirth. Talk to each other about how you would deal with a baby who is deformed or a baby who is stillborn. Pregnancy forces you to look at all the possibilities and to discuss what you would do in such an event. I say this not to focus on any of the negative possibilities—but to prepare you.

When I think about childbirth, I like to remember how another culture views it. In Africa, the woman who is in labor is seen as having to cross a fast and rushing river. She must walk across the river alone on a narrow log; although she can have help from either side. People in canoes may assist her to stay on the log. If she slips, they can help her up again. There are women waiting on the other side of the banks; they have already taken this journey.

Each woman must take this voyage alone. But as the coach, you can be there for her to keep her from going under, pulled by the fast rushing currents within her body. Remind her to let you know what works and what doesn't. Her feedback is your best guide. It may help to consider what you both would like the labor to be. Write down some personal affirmations on the subject. Examples of such affirmations would be:

○ I am willing to let my body surrender to the opening process of labor. I will do my best to relax and flow with the process.

○ As a coach I am willing to observe and guide you to the best of my ability, helping to make your labor as relaxed an experience as possible.

○ I accept the perfect works of my body to let this baby out into the universe, healthily and safely.

Let your affirmations express your positive sentiments about the birth.

Having a baby is an incredible, wonderful process. The more you involve yourself in the preparation and the actual birth, the richer it is for you and the foundation of your family. If you talk with a man who has experienced his child's birth, he'll tell you he wouldn't have missed it for anything on earth. It is special. So are you. Your guidance and presence as a coach/partner are something you will never forget.

A CRIB SHEET FOR COACHES: LABOR AND REVIEW

In spite of all your practice, you may get forgetful in the excitement of the real thing. I have therefore included a quick and easy chart to help coaches review, at a glance, possible techniques and when they might be most useful. Have a Xerox copy made and save it to use as a crib sheet in the hospital. Don't feel limited by any of the suggestions. If you come up with something that works, use it. If you'd care to share your discoveries with me, I'd be delighted. Write me and let me know what you've found. My address is in the Resource Guide at the back of the book.

LABOR REVIEW SHEET

Stage One: Beginning Signs

o May have bloody show (loss of mucous plug).
o Rupture of membranes.
o May have bloody show (loss of mucous plug).
o Rupture of membranes.
o Intermittent backache.
o Diarrhea.
o Contractions; regular or irregular, becoming closer together and more intense.
o 8–10 hours for complete effacement.
o 0–4 centimeters = first stage, contractions are 5–20 minutes apart and are 30–60 seconds duration.

Laboring Mother

o Sleep, rest, relax.
o Hot bath; if membranes have ruptured, shower only.
o Tea with honey.
o May eat lightly if hungry.
o Fruit, broth, juice, water okay.
o Slow, relaxed abdominal breathing.
o Relax pelvic floor.
o Have an enema.
o Relax and enjoy the beginning of labor.

Coach

o Make sure everything is ready for your birth experience.
o Help her with the enema.
o *Be there!* Give emotional and verbal support.
o Time contractions periodically, noting *Duration* (from beginning to end) and *Frequency* (from beginning to beginning).
o Report rupture to doctor.
o Remind her to urinate every hour.
o If membranes rupture wash area after each bowel movement.
o Use massage, touch, music, baths (if the water hasn't broken) to aid body relaxation.
o Don't let her become too active.

LABOR REVIEW SHEET

Active Phase

- 3–5 hours in length.
- 4–8 centimenters dilation.
- Contractions 2–5 minutes apart.
- 45–50 seconds duration.
- May have backache, cold feet, leg pains, discomfort in lower abdomen.
- Need for coach to be very close by.

Laboring Mother

- Slow, relaxed abdominal breathing; may speed up during height of contraction.
- Follow your body rhythms.
- Deep cleansing breaths between contractions.
- Relax perineum.
- May need to squat or use knee-chest position if backache present; do *Pelvic Rocks* between contractions.

Coach

- Time-distortion techniques: rest, pleasure, labor completion.
- Breathe with her if necessary.
- Soft soothing voice can help to relax.
- Remind her to urinate.
- Help with cool, wet wash cloths.
- Back and leg massage.
- Counterpressure to back during contractions.
- Suggest positions if there is back labor.
- *Give encouragement.*
- Do not leave after 6 centimeters.
- Massage perineum with oil.

Transition

- ½–2 hours in length.
- 8–10 centimeters dilation.
- 60–90 seconds in duration.
- 1-minute intervals; long peak.
- *They do not get stronger!*

Laboring Mother

- *Slow, relaxed breathing* when able.
- Blowing at peak (speeding up then slowing down again).
- Deep cleansing breaths between contractions.

Coach

- Coach breathing; help her to slow down when able.
- *Be positive, loving, encouraging.*
- Talk about baby coming soon, tell her what a good job she's doing.

LABOR REVIEW SHEET

Transition (cont.)

○ Concentration directed and centered.
○ May have bloody show; an urge to push.
○ Signs: Change in mood; no time between contractions, may experience chills, trembling, belching or nausea, rectal pressure.
○ Rupture of membranes.

Laboring Mother

○ If urge to push before fully dilated, *blow, blow, blow* (slowly); open mouth and relax bottom or breathe slowly.

Coach

○ Help to avoid hyperventilation—keep her breathing slowly.
○ Offer cool washcloths.
○ If not fully dilated, if she has urge to push, *help her to blow, blow, blow,* slowly.
○ Use hot compresses to ease any perineum stretching and prevent tearing.

Stage Two: Birth

○ Lasts ½–2 hours.
○ Contractions easier to control.
○ 2–4 minutes apart.
○ Last 60 seconds.
○ Strong urge to push.
○ Active pushing— feels good!
○ New energy.
○ Feel baby's head in birth canal.
○ Vaginal and perineal muscles stretching.
○ Perineal massage.
○ Hot packs.

Laboring Mother

○ Expulsion Techniques:
Two cleansing breaths. Inhale, chin on chest. Bear down and out. Relax pelvic floor, feet, legs.
Hold breath for count of 10, exhale, tilt head back, inhale lightly, resume pushing.
○ Relax between contractions with cleansing breaths.
○ When told to stop pushing, *blow, blow, blow* to control urge.
○ Feel baby's head when crowning.

Coach

○ Move to the Delivery Room.
○ Make sure she is elevated and has lots of pillows.
○ If possible, sit behind her during pushing.
○ Provide support and comfort.
○ Remind her to put her chin on her chest.
○ Help her hold her breath by counting to 10 backwards.
○ Help her relax pelvic floor, thighs, and feet.
○ Expect the baby's head to be delivered slowly.
○ Help her blow when asked to stop pushing.

137

LABOR REVIEW SHEET

Expulsion of Placenta	*Laboring Mother*	*Coach*
○ Cord is cut. ○ Placenta, membranes, cord are delivered. ○ Stitches if necessary. ○ Baby covered with vernix. ○ Baby may be slightly blue but will pink up. ○ Sometimes syringe for mucus in throat.	○ Touch baby; massage back and head. ○ Drop in metabolic rate produces a chill. ○ Sometimes trembling. ○ May feel a few more contractions, then *push* placenta out. ○ Sometimes contractions when baby nurses. ○ May be hungry, tired, but totally fulfilled and full of energy. *You've worked hard and done a good job. Congratulations, Mom!!*	○ Touch baby; massage its back and head. ○ Make sure mother gets juice to drink. ○ One for you too! *You have worked hard and deserve praise. Congratulations, coach!*

4. A look within: the anatomy of pregnancy, labor, and delivery

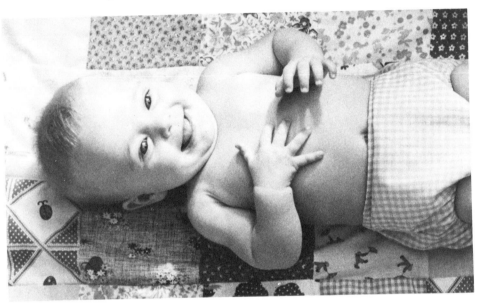

This chapter grew from a desire to witness what goes on inside the mother. How does the baby grow and develop? Most women have no idea what their vagina looks like, let alone the vaginal muscular structure. What better time and place to learn than while you are pregnant? There is also a section in this chapter on the process of labor and delivery. This section will illustrate the stages that were discussed in Chapter 3 and will prepare you to understand, from the inside, what you will be seeing in Chapter 5—the photo essays of two births.

When I was pregnant, I wanted to see what the baby looked like during different phases. The following drawings serve as a reminder of our amazing capacity to nurture and create life within us.

FETAL DEVELOPMENT

Fertilization and Implantation of the Egg

First a mature egg is released from the ovary and enters the Fallopian tube. There it is met by the sperm and in this case fertilized. Next, the fertilized egg travels through the tube to the uterus. It implants in the lining around the seventh day. At this time it is a round ball of approximately 150 cells.

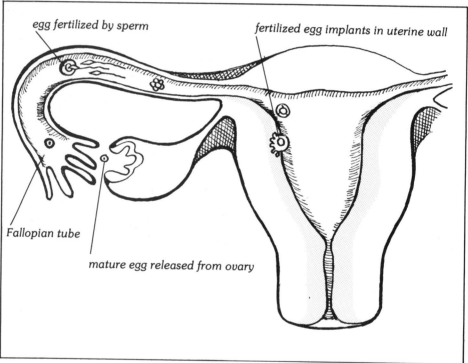

Fertilization and implantation of the egg

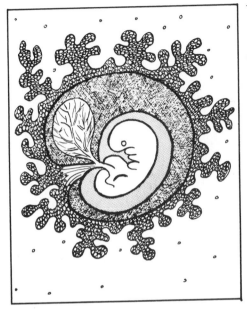
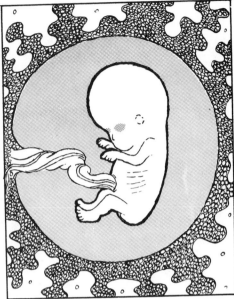

Embryo at 4 weeks: 3/16th of an inch   *Embryo at 8 weeks: 1 inch long*

Embryo at 4 Weeks: 3/16 of an inch

In one month the fertilized egg has grown 10,000 times the size of its first cells. The placenta, now the yolk sack, is beginning to form. You can see the buds for the arms and legs. The mouth, lower jaw, and throat are now developing. The backbone and spinal column are forming. The heart can beat 65 times a minute.

Embryo at 8 Weeks: 1 inch long

The face and features are forming. The limbs are beginning to show distinct divisions into arms and leg parts. The long bones and internal organs are developing. Teeth are being formed.

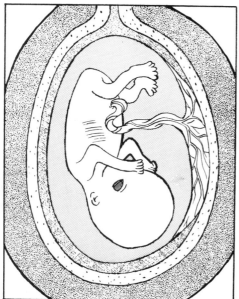 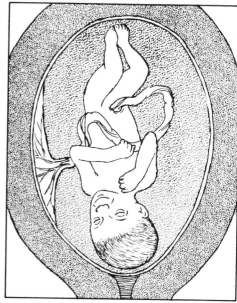

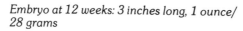

Embryo at 12 weeks: 3 inches long, 1 ounce/ 28 grams

Fetus at 16 weeks: 6–8 inches long, 6 ounces/168 grams

Embryo at 12 Weeks: 3 inches long, 1 ounce/28 grams

The basic structure is finished. The fingernails and toenails are beginning to develop. Primitive hair follicles are forming and so are the beginning of the vocal cords.

Fetus at 16 Weeks: 6–8 inches long, 6 ounces/168 grams

Now called a fetus, it can move freely, has a strong heartbeat, fair digestion, and active muscles. The placenta is almost fully developed. Lanugo (a fine hair) is beginning to cover the body. The brain is like a miniature adult's. Sweat glands are forming and the skin is thickening into various layers.

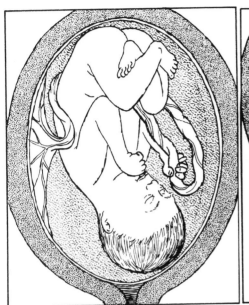
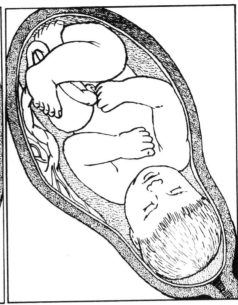

Fetus at 24 weeks: 14 inches long, 18 ounces/504 grams

Baby at term—38–42 weeks: 19–22 inches long, 6–9 pounds/3–4 kilograms

Fetus at 24 Weeks: 14 inches long, 18 ounces/504 grams

Mother has felt quickening, the baby's movement. Buds of the second teeth have grown under the first set. Internal organs are maturing rapidly. Vernix (a white cheeselike coating) is developing to protect the skin. The eyes are open and sensitive to light. The baby can now hear sounds.

Baby at Term—38–42 Weeks: 19–22 inches long, 6–9 pounds/3–4 kilograms

Only the downy hair on the arms and shoulders remains. The lungs are now fully developed. The baby is complete, ready to be born!

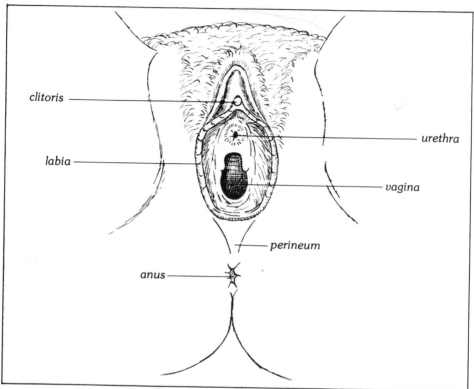

Pelvic floor from the outside

THE PELVIC FLOOR

Many pregnant women become very curious about what their genitals look like. This drawing shows the external parts of the vagina. It also explains why the perineum, because of its central position, is such a key focus during birth. It must relax and stretch to let the baby out. Because of the increase in fluids and hormones during childbirth, it can stretch an amazing distance.

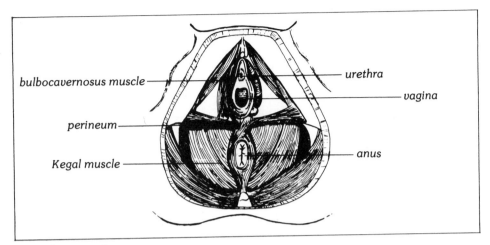

Pelvic floor muscles

We have a very intricate system of muscles supporting our vagina and rectum. When the baby is pushed out, the muscles surrounding the vaginal opening, the bulbocavernosus muscle, must also relax and stretch. This drawing shows what the muscles that "feed" into the perineum look like.

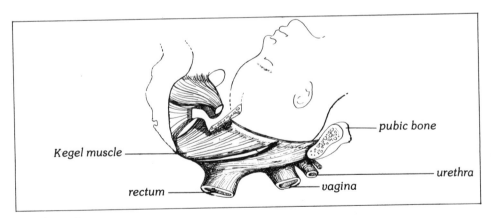

Kegel muscle

The muscle below the baby's head (the pelvic floor muscle) is called the "kegel" or the pubococcygeus muscle. It extends from the pubic bone to the coccyx or tailbone. This drawing helped me understand how critical the kegel muscle is in guiding the baby's head out the birth canal during labor. It also let me see how important it is to do the kegel exercise daily to help (1) recognize where it is, and (2) know how to relax it during labor. In later life, a well-toned kegel muscle prevents prolapsing.

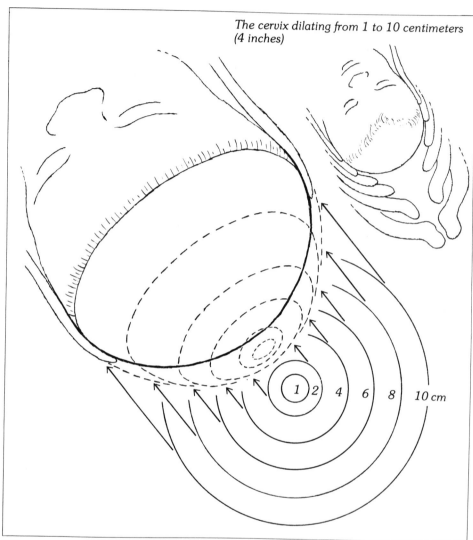

The cervix dilating from 1 to 10 centimeters (4 inches)

Effacement and dilation of the cervix

THE FIRST STAGE OF LABOR

As labor begins, the cervix effaces (thins out).

Effacement is followed by a gradual dilation (stretching open) of the cervix from 1 to 10 centimeters (4 inches).

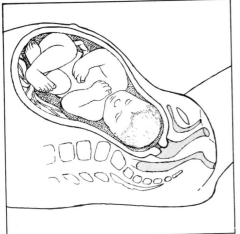
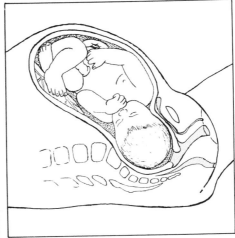

Onset of labor

Active phase

LABOR AND DELIVERY

Onset of Labor

The first stage begins with the thinning or effacing of the cervix. Effacement can occur silently, or for some women, be a cramping or twinging sensation.

Active Phase

Next, the cervix will begin to dilate, or stretch open. It is very important to keep the bladder and rectum clear. You might want to have an enema now, early in labor.

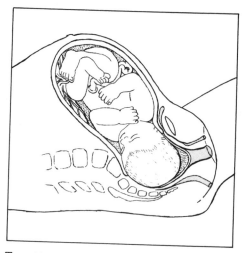

Transition—completion of first stage

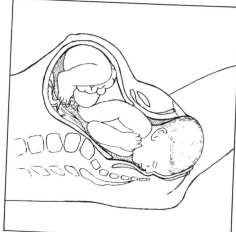

Second stage—pushing

Transition: Completion of first stage

The cervix completes its dilation from 7 to 10 centimeters. Often rectal pressure is felt strongly. Don't push yet. Contractions are longer and more intense. This is the shortest stage of labor and requires the most concentrated attention from support people.

Second stage: Pushing

Once the "hatch door" is opened completely, you will start to push the baby out. Its head is built to mold and thus fit through the birth canal. As the head starts to push out, avoid actively pushing. Breathe the head out.

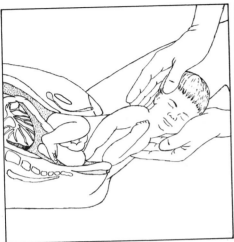

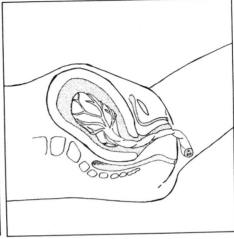

The baby is born!   *Third stage: expulsion of the placenta*

The Baby Is Born!

After the head is out, it will rotate to the side. This is called *restitution*. The shoulders and body will follow. You will see what took nine months to nurture and create.

Third stage: Expulsion of the placenta

The placenta, which has completed its function of nourishing the baby, must now be pushed out entirely. This is vital to the mother's health and recovery. The uterus can then return to a nonpregnant state.

5. *Two births: photo essays*

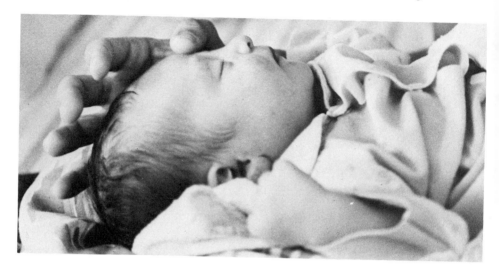

We are living in a time of many exciting birth choices. Women can now choose to go to hospitals, have their babies at birth centers, or even deliver at home. When I became pregnant I knew I would give birth at home, so I diligently set out to find information and a midwife. Home birth is not for everyone. What is important is that you feel comfortable with your choice and that you take full responsibility for your decision.

In this chapter you will see two birth experiences: my daughter's home birth, and Tiffany's hospital birth. Each birth has its own unique story yet illuminates a common theme. Both Susan and I prepared for our labor with prenatal exercises. Here is a documentary of how these exercises helped our labors.

BIRTH 1: ANNA'S BIRTH

My labor began at three in the morning with contractions starting three minutes apart. Bob was a wonderful coach and a great masseur. As labor picked up I found different positions comfortable. I was glad that I had practiced sitting like this (*Mountain Pose*). It really helped as the contractions got stronger.

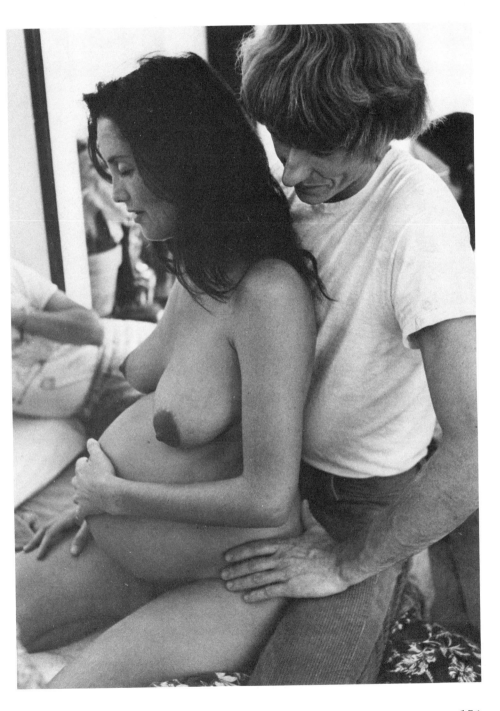

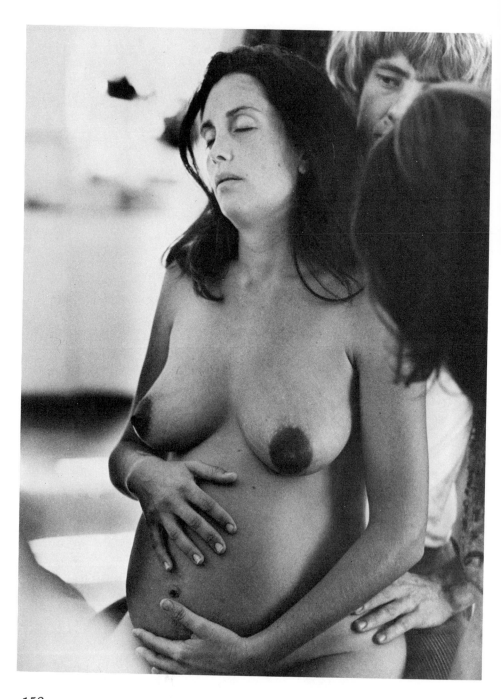

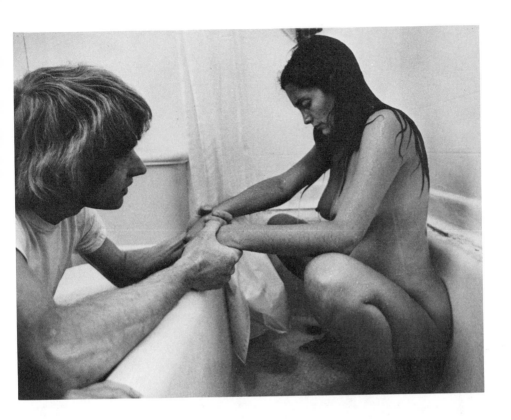

Breathing techniques became essential. I found slow abdominal breathing the most useful. It helped me to concentrate and eased the tension in my body. I also found lightly rubbing my belly to be relaxing.

Right before transition, I fell asleep. After I had napped for 45 minutes, the midwife suggested I get up and take a shower. It was 95 degrees outside and the thought of cold water was irresistible. Labor picked up in the shower. Squatting during a contraction helped me feel centered and grounded (*Squatting Breath*).

Walking and taking the shower had helped my labor get started again, only now it was all back labor. The hard part of the baby's head was pressing against the hard part of my sacrum. Leaning forward (*The Turtle* pose) helped move the head off my spine.

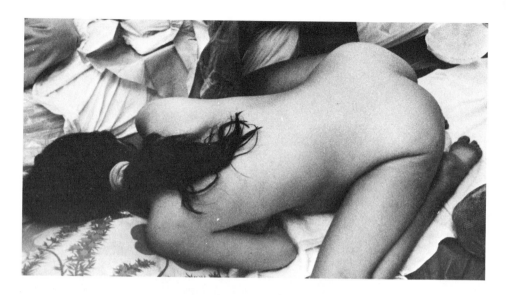

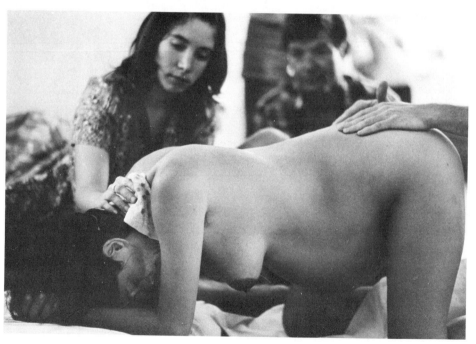

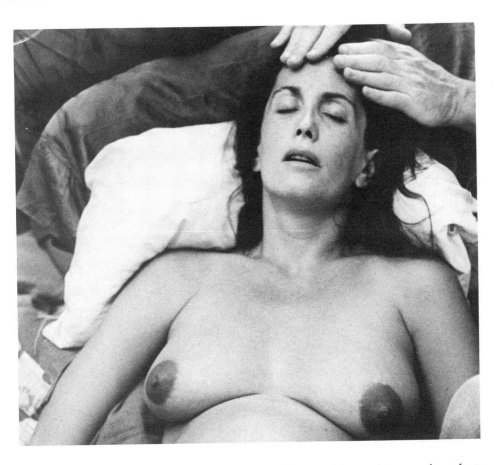

I attempted to turn the baby's head around by rocking my hips from side to side (*Pelvic Rock*) and then coming into a squatting position between contractions to maintain the progress made by the rocking. It worked!

My body was now dilated to 10 centimeters and I was ready to push. At first I tensed my shoulders and clenched my jaw, but I soon got the knack and was able to sit back and relax more. The baby's head had definitely made progress and I felt a great sense of relief (*Kingdom Gates*).

Somewhere from the middle of my being came the energy for the loudest roar I have ever made. There was no tension, just pure pushing and roaring. What a glorious feeling. Opening my mouth and relaxing helped my vagina open too.

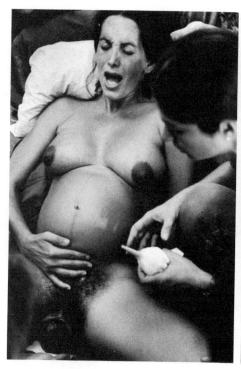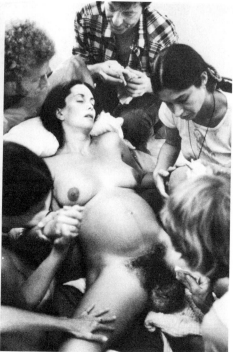

We could see the head at last. The stinging I had felt around the lips of my vagina was gone. In the next push or two I would see the baby I had worked nine months to nurture and create.

When the shoulders had cleared I couldn't wait to reach down and guide my baby out. I wanted her *now*. She opened her eyes as soon as her head turned. She wanted to see her new world.

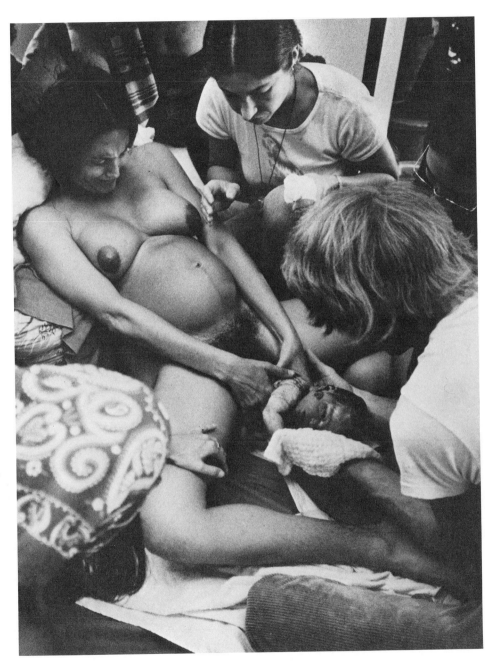

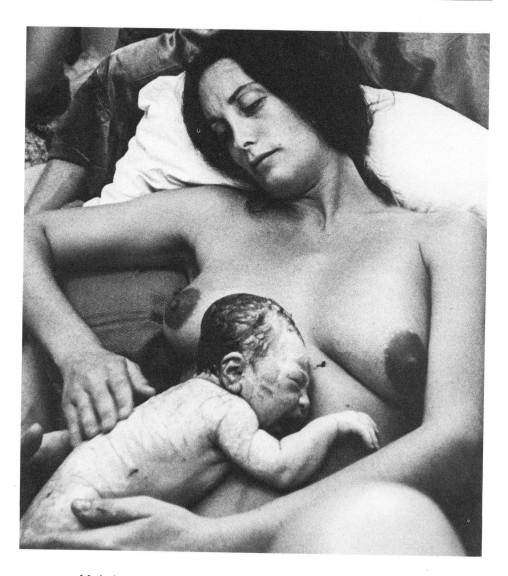

My baby arrived ten days early and was covered with vernix. Notice how her head is molded. She looked beautiful to me.

Less than 24 hours later, here we are together. My labor had lasted 12 hours; then Anna and I had fallen asleep together. The molding on her head has gone down quite a bit already. I felt so wonderful to see my daughter's healthy little body-spirit. Welcome, Anna Rachael!

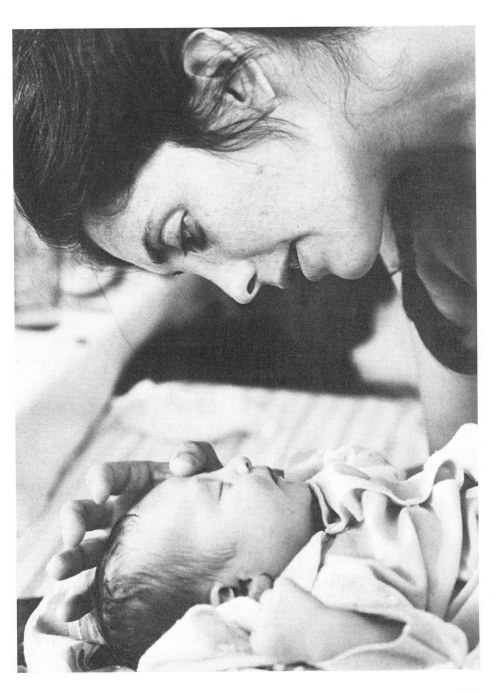

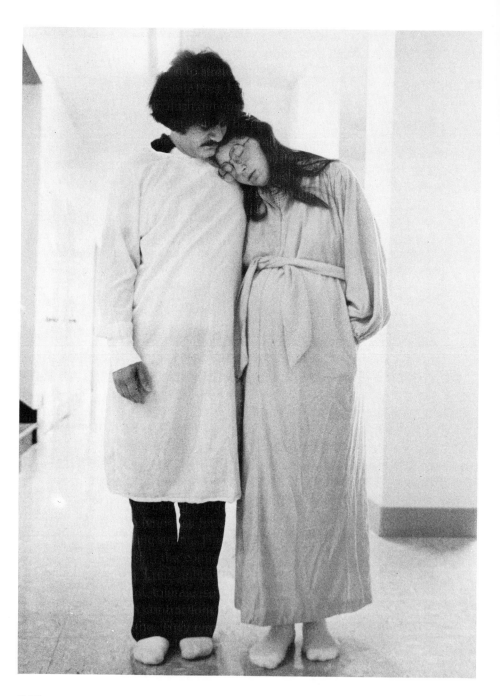

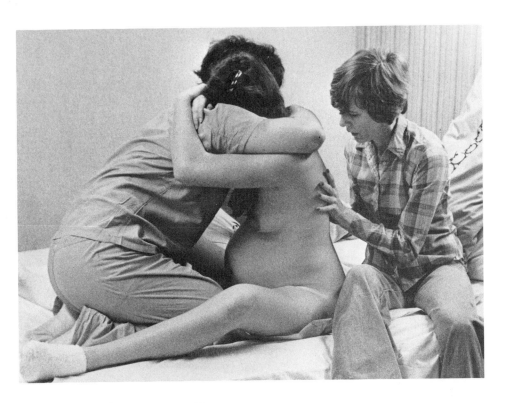

BIRTH 2: TIFFANY'S BIRTH

Susan and Doug decided on a hospital birth. The following pages record the birth of their daughter at California's Hollywood Presbyterian Medical Center.

Susan arrived at the Center at 12:00 in the afternoon. She was dilated to 3 centimeters. As her labor was progressing slowly, she and Doug started to walk up and down the corridor. Here she is having a contraction. Walking helped pick up the tempo of the labor. In fact, Susan felt better walking than lying down.

Her labor began in the Medical Center's Alternative Birth Center, whose rooms have double beds. This allowed Susan to get support by holding and hugging Doug while her mother gave helpful massage.

161

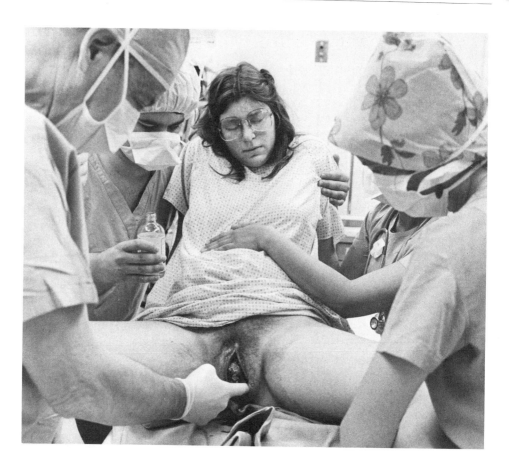

Labor was progressing slowly, about 1 centimeter every three hours, and she was very tired, so Susan's doctor decided to transfer her out of the Alternative Birth Center. With the help of a pitocin drip, labor picked up. Vaginal massage and hot compresses helped her perineum stretch. During the delivery, the doctor was a delight to watch. He continued to massage the vaginal walls with oil and allowed Susan to sit up without the use of stirrups or the clutter of sterile drapes on her legs. She was relieved to be able to deliver in this manner (*Kingdom Gates*).

One last push and into the world for Tiffany. The doctor let the baby slide gently into his hands. There was no pulling, pushing, twisting, or episiotomy. Thanks to the massage and hot compresses, Susan didn't tear.

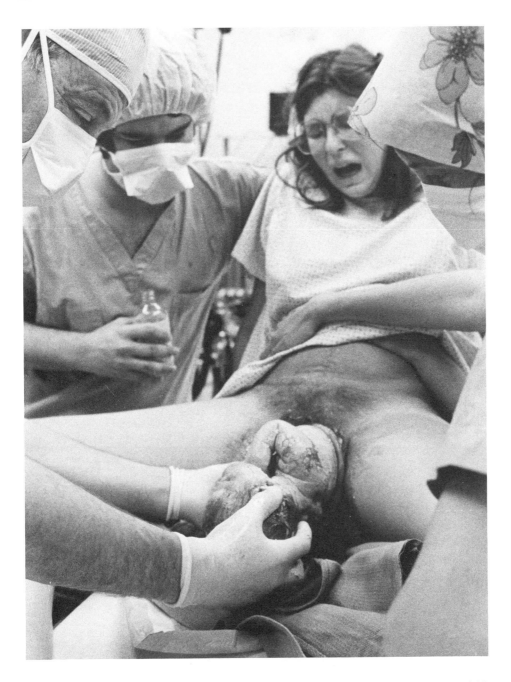

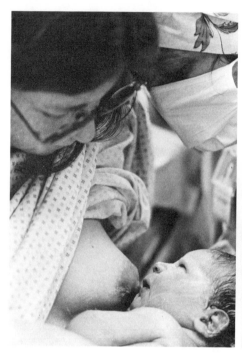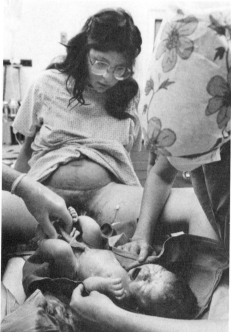

Tiffany went right to her mother's breast. This was their first chance to really look at each other.

After the cord stopped pulsating, it was clamped. Doug was allowed to cut it. Tiffany was wiped off a bit, then given to her father to hold. She weighed in at 7 pounds, 3 ounces, 20 inches long—a respectable size for a first baby!

The placenta was delivered, so Susan could now lie down and relax. The nurses got the water ready to give Tiffany a bath. The tub was wheeled close to Susan's bed so that she could join Doug in this ritual.

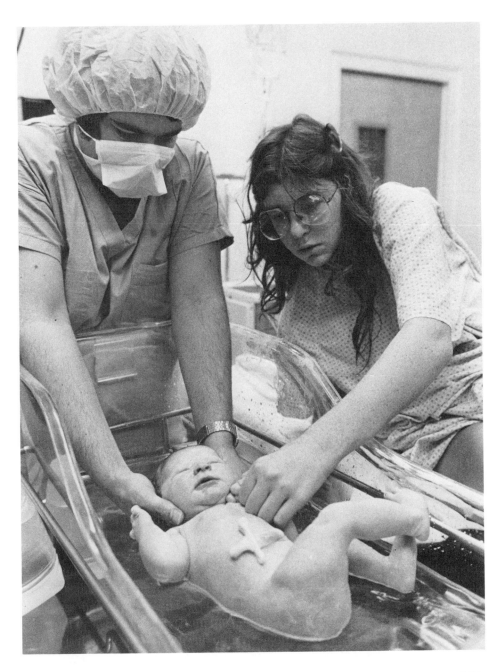

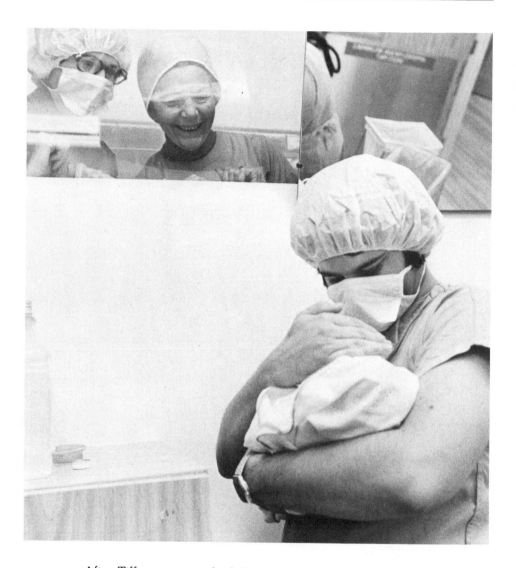

  After Tiffany was washed, Doug walked her over to the observation window. Susan's mother and grandmother, who had been at the hospital all night, were thrilled to see the new baby.

  The new family was taken to the postpartum recovery room. Susan and Doug stayed with Tiffany for an hour and Susan was able to nurse her there. Labor had lasted 18 hours, but now it was over. Congratulations, Mom and Dad—welcome, Tiffany!

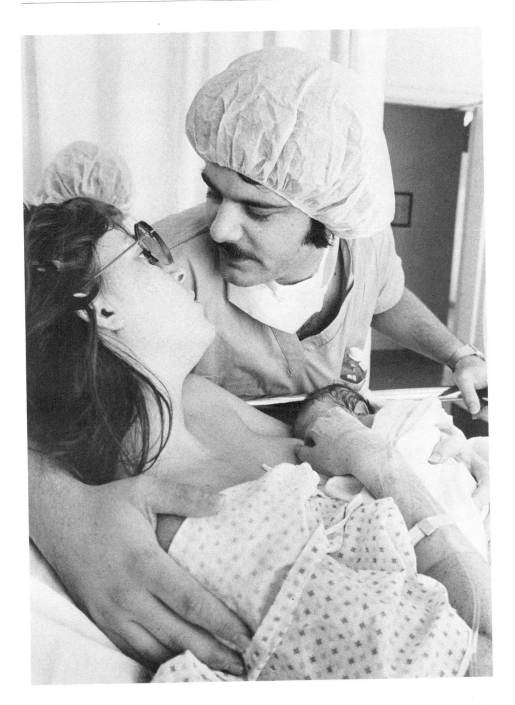

6. *Postpartum exercises*

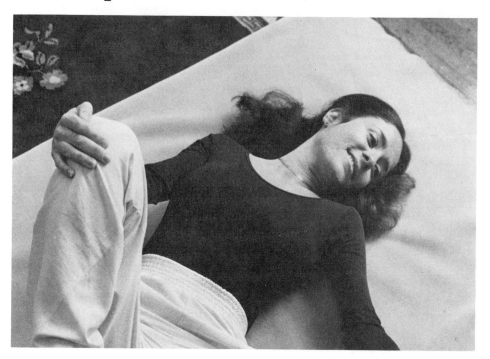

You have just participated in the miracle of birth, one of life's profoundest experiences. You are now entering a whole new phase of your life—motherhood. This postpartum period is a time rich in reward and discovery but it is a time of adjustment, too. You will be learning all about your baby; you will be coping with your new role as a parent; you will be getting in touch with your changed body. One of the best ways to get back in tune with yourself is through movement. Proper exercise during the six weeks following birth can both enhance the postpartum period and speed your recovery.

You may ask yourself: Can I exercise right away? Which exercises are safe to do? Where will I find time to exercise now that I am so busy with the baby? These are all perfectly natural questions. The first step is to look at yourself and see what condition your body is in. Stand in front of a mirror. Notice what you like and dislike about your body. In what ways is it the same as before your pregnancy? How and where is it different?

Now close your eyes and visualize yourself moving. Try to see every part of your body. After a few moments, stop imagining and actually move around for a few minutes. Don't think about it. Just move. Feel where you want to or need to stretch, and move accordingly. This is what exercise is: movement set down in ritualized form to be repeated and shared by others.

Postnatal exercise is not just for Mom. Recently a great deal of attention has been focused on the importance of touching and moving newborn babies. Dr. Frederick LeBoyer, in *Birth Without Violence*, reminds us of the importance of a gentle, quiet birth. Marshall Klauss and J. Kennell's work (e.g. "Human Maternal Behavior at first contact with their young." *Pediatrics,* 1970, 46[2]) stresses the importance of holding and bonding with the newborn. Ashley Montagu, in his book *Touching*, emphasizes the comfort in nurturing through touch. Exercising with your baby is a close, loving process for both of you. It helps give babies a sense of their body and how it can work. You are also helping to set up an early pattern of confidence between you and your child. You know how she or he moves because you have been an integral part of the child's motor development.

In Chapters 7 and 8 we will look at exercises Mom and Dad can do with the baby. This chapter is devoted to the new mother. It is divided into two sections: postnatal exercises for Mom during the first six weeks, and special information and exercises for Cesarean mothers.

SETTING THE STAGE

The better your frame of mind when you exercise, the more you will profit from your movements. Here are some tips on how to eliminate stress from your daily life during the early postpartum weeks, thereby giving your body maximum opportunity to rest and recover.

Establishing Priorities

When you are a mother, time becomes a critical factor. How do you find enough of it? You feed, change, and bathe the baby and half the day is gone. True, you are moving at a much slower pace. Accept this and relax. Time does open up. By developing a schedule, you will be able to do most of what you want to accomplish.

The key to solving time problems is to organize your activities in accord with your desires. What do you most *want* to do? Write your preferences down, and then cross off the things on your list that you don't feel are essential.

When you block out your day, don't forget to leave time to do a few things for yourself. It may be a shower or a walk around the block, but *do* it. Remember, you are important. Be sure to leave time to rest. Take frequent naps with your baby. If you are tired you won't be able to enjoy anything. You'll be cranky, tired, fussy, and a difficult person to be around. But if you are in good health and good spirits, you will approach your family, chores, and life in a way that is beneficial to all concerned.

Accepting Help and Support

Since one of your main jobs during these first six weeks is to rest, let your friends lend a hand. If they want to cook, clean, or share the housework, permit them to pitch in. Company makes homemaking faster and much more enjoyable. Friends like to rally to the aid of a new mother.

Plan to have time alone, other than when the baby is sleeping. Arrange to leave the baby with your husband or a friend for even an hour. I can't stress this enough. You need time to yourself, even if it is only for a brief period. It will enhance your entire experience as a mother, woman, person.

If you feel you need outside support, get in touch with people from your childbirth class. They will have new babies too. If you are having problems breastfeeding, or simply want to share your experiences, contact the La Leche League (see the Resource Guide at the back of the book) and go to their meetings. Your childbirth teacher may know of other local support groups where you can meet other mothers who are experiencing situations similar to yours. Remember, you are not alone.

To Relieve Engorged (Overfilled with Milk) Breasts

This can be a problem for *all* new mothers.
○ Ask the nurse to teach you how to hand express your milk.
○ If your baby is unavailable for nursing, you can hand express colostrum and have the baby drink it from a bottle. This will help clear up any breast engorgement and give the baby a fine source of sustenance. Some babies and mothers need to

nurse more often than every four hours. Ask the nurses to bring your baby more frequently.

o Sometimes wearing a breast cup can help prevent engorgement.

o Use very warm washcloths or compresses to get the milk flowing. If you can take a shower or soak your breasts in a bowl of warm water, you can often get the milk to flow right out.

Many of these exercises were described in detail in Chapter 2. As a brief reminder, here are short descriptions of them, as well as some new ones. Start with the first exercise and then add one a day onto your exercise routine. Increase the number of times gradually.

POSTNATAL EXERCISES FOR THE FIRST SIX WEEKS

The following exercises are designed to help you recover from childbirth easily and with more energy. When you feel an ache, then stretch, breathe, and move. If you're not ready to exercise yet, don't waste time feeling guilty. It took me three months to establish a regular home exercise program for me and my daughter.

Before you begin the exercises, review the exercise tips at the beginning of Chapter 2. They still apply. Since most of these new exercises are modifications of the ones you did when you were pregnant, redesigned to meet your new needs, they should be easier now. You are familiar with them and your muscles share that memory. You will be less likely to strain or feel tense as you move.

Start slowly and build up gradually. Whenever you feel any stress, *stop*. These exercises can feel good. The more you enjoy them, the more you will want to exercise.

Breathing

Alternate Nostril Breathing: Close your left nostril, inhale through the right, open the left nostril and exhale (closing the right); inhale through the left side, open the right side to exhale, continue alternating.

Abdominal Breathing: Your abdomen expands as you inhale and presses in on the exhale—a low, slow gradual breathing.

Costal Breathing: On each inhalation, expand your rib cage out to the sides; exhale and let your rib cage relax.

Candle-Blowing Breath: Gently push the air out your mouth; let the inhalation happen automatically, focus on the exhalation.

All of the above breathing styles relax and tone the muscles around your rib cage, abdomen, and diaphragm. When I first started nursing, I realized my nipples were not as prepared as I had thought. Abdominal breathing helped me relax and nurse Anna with much less discomfort.

Day 1 - Kegel Exercise

The importance of this exercise after childbirth cannot be sufficiently stressed. Now when you do this exercise, focus on tightening your vaginal muscles instead of relaxing the muscles. Count to five as you tighten the muscle, then count to four as you slowly release. This routine can help you control your bladder during the first weeks after birth and, more important, can help avoid any prolapsing later on. The *Kegel* can be a friend of yours for the rest of your life. Teach it to your daughter also. In many cultures it is a matter of course to instruct young girls how to tone their vaginal muscle. Your pelvic floor needs to maintain tone just as your stomach and legs do.

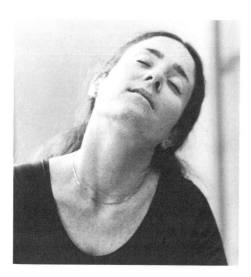

Day 2 - Head and Neck Rolls

Let your head drop forward and make slow circles in one direction, stop and reverse the direction. Let your shoulders stay as still as possible. These movements are a blessing for a nursing mother. They help relieve the tension you get from nursing and holding your baby six to eight hours a day. *Head and Neck Rolls* can be done sitting in bed the day after you deliver.

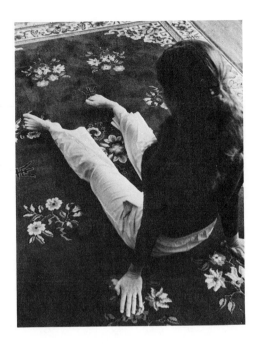

Day 3 - Ankle Works

Lie down or sit up and roll your ankles in one direction, then the other. Press the balls of your feet forward and then press your heels forward to stretch your calf and shin muscles.

You probably won't be walking around much at first. Your legs, however, will want attention. To help the circulation to your feet and legs, you can start the ankle rolls and movements on the third day after you deliver.

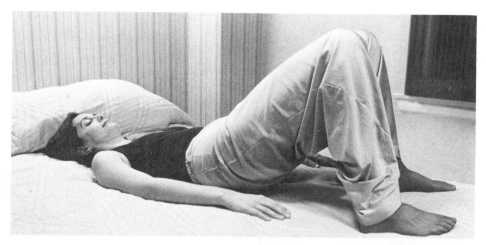

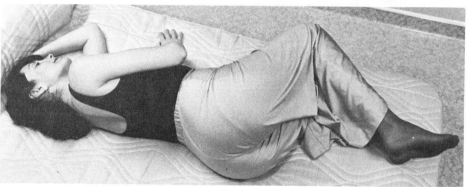

Day 4 - Pelvis Rocking

Lie on your back, knees down flat on the bed or floor. Press the small of your back into the floor, and barely lift your bottom off the bed (floor). Hold for a moment, then inhale and slowly return your buttocks to the bed (floor). Establish an easy rocking motion with a slight pause in the middle. You might also try a variation, lying on your side. Tuck and arch your lower back gently. This movement helps to stimulate intestinal activity without your standing up. If you want to do the *Pelvic Rocks*, the way you did them when you were pregnant, wait at least a week, possibly two, depending on how you feel.

174

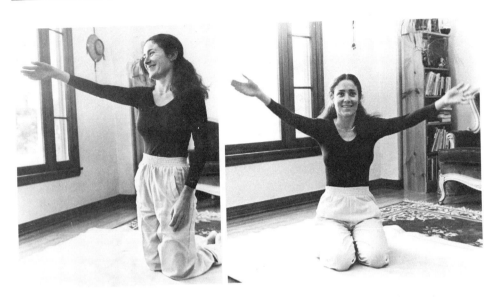

Day 5 - Arm Circles

Stand or sit and circle one arm, inhaling. Exhale as you swing your arm in the opposite direction.

Although *Arm Circles* don't feel strenuous, you should take it easy for the first month. Then you can graduate to the *Milkmaid*.

Milkmaid

Both palms face forward. Make large circles in one direction, then reverse the direction. Make the circles gently and with as little effort as possible. Be patient: you will be moving up to full steam in a few weeks; don't try to push yourself too early.

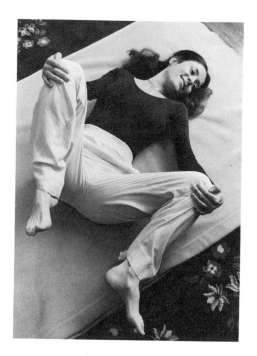

Day 6 - The Cradle

Lie on your back. Hold each knee to the chest and roll to one side. Lift and open the top leg, roll over to the other side, and continue rolling slowly from side to side. For tight or stiff backs this exercise can feel wonderful. Your inner thighs will hum from the gentle stretch. I still love to do this one. By the end of the first week you can easily add this to your exercise routine.

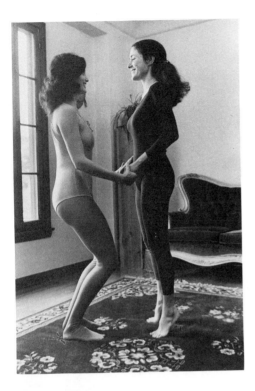

Day 7 - Elevator

Stand with your feet parallel, slowly rise up onto the balls of your feet. Lower your heels. Now bend your knees, but keep your heels on the ground. After about a week of good rest, your legs will want some retoning. This exercise from your pregnancy will help your ankles, calves, and thighs gather strength through gentle activity. This exercise is fun to do holding the baby to whom it feels like an elevator ride.

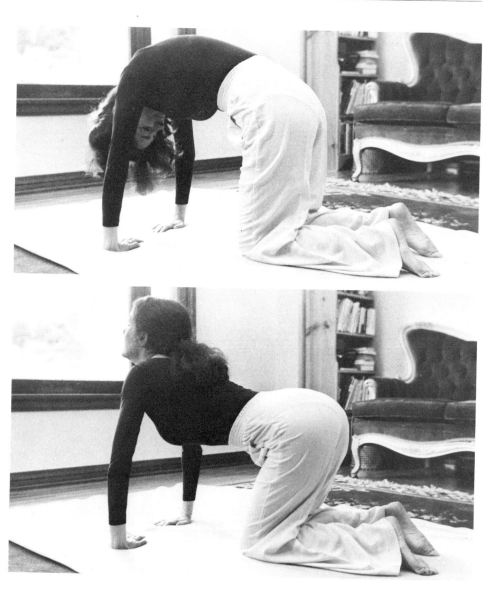

Day 8 - Pelvic Rocks

On your hands and knees, tuck your pelvis under while you arch your back and tuck your head down, stretching your neck. Next, let your back relax and sway, letting your chin stretch up. Continue arching and swaying. This is the best exercise for lower back problems. I found that after carrying my daughter around for a few hours, I needed some relief for my lower back muscles.

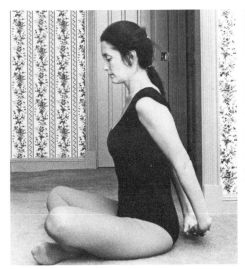 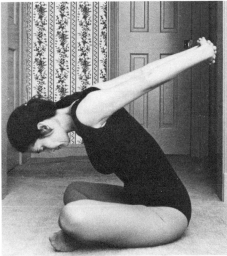

Day 9 - Nursing Stretch

Sit with your legs tucked under your buttocks. Clasp your hands behind your back. Raise your hands as you lean forward. Lift your arms as high as you can. Go as far forward as you can, until the top of your head touches the floor. Gently rock your body forward and back, stop. Lift your head off the floor, sit up but keep your arms as far away from your body as you can. Once you are sitting back on your heels, let your hands float apart.

Nursing tends to shorten the muscles in our chest, called the pectoral muscles. We tend to hunch our shoulders forward and this can create soreness or stiffness. This exercise is a blessing for all nursing mothers. Stretching your neck and rocking gently back and forth on the top of your head helps to open those muscles, as well as improve circulation to your head.

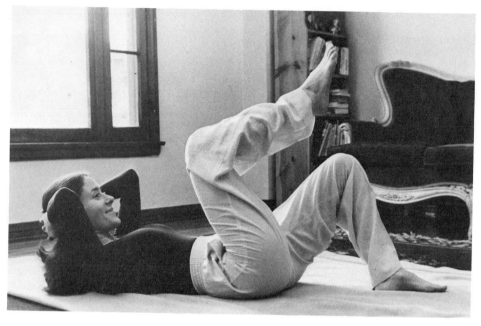

Day 10 - Knee Circles

Lie on your back. Bend one knee, with foot on the floor. Lift the other foot off the floor, bending your knee, and gently draw circles in the air with your knee. Reverse the direction. Rest your knee after fully exploring the range of your knee's movements. Reverse sides. (If you keep your knee bent, you can fully explore the range of movement in your hip socket without straining your lower back.)

Allow yourself to be playful. I like to trace out the letters of the alphabet in the air with my knee or foot. Sometimes I even draw pictures. Put on some music and vary the rhythm. Let your leg dance!

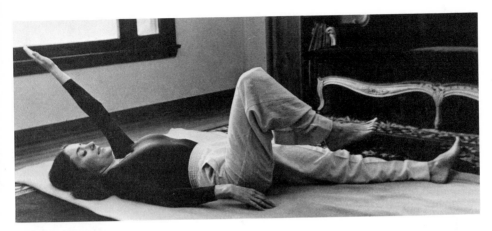

Day 11 - Cross Crawling

Lie on your back. Lift your right knee and your left arm at the same time. Bring your knee toward your abdomen while you are raising your arm over your head. Lower your arm and leg together. Repeat on the other side, raising your left knee and your right arm. Continue alternating sides. Remember to breathe. You will benefit from doing this exercise, and, as you will see in the next chapter, your baby will too. It helps to balance your body's energy between your right and left sides. Start to do a few of these in the morning before you get out of bed on the tenth or eleventh day after delivery. Don't force any of the movements. Let your knee and wrist feel as if there are strings attached to each one, gently lifting and lowering. Lift only as high as is comfortable for you. Don't try to reach any goal. Your body benefits from the experience and awareness of each movement.

At this point in your exercise program, you should be nearing the end of your second week. Vary the order and increase the number of times you do each of the above exercises. Keep in mind that your system took nine months to build a baby; it will take about that long to return to shape.

Your intestines were quite cramped by the end of your pregnancy. That is one of the reasons you want to be gentle with yourself now. They take about six weeks to return to their original space. Another spot that is healing is the lining of your uterus where the placenta was attached. You will have a discharge for about six weeks, called lochia, which gradually disappears. Initially lochia is red and gradually becomes brownish—like a menstrual cycle. If you notice any *bright* red bleeding, you have engaged in activity that is too strenuous for your body at that time. Stop, breathe, relax, and wait. You will be able to resume a full and active life soon, but not quite yet. Whenever you take a new activity back into your schedule, notice how you feel. If you experience any light-headedness, stop. Remember that you have just given birth. You need time to recover from this important and strenuous event.

SPECIAL INFORMATION AND EXERCISES FOR CESAREAN MOMS

With the rise in Cesarean operations in this country (between 10 and 40 percent, depending on the hospital), a special section for Cesarean mothers is essential. This part of the book contains comfort measures and safe exercises for those of you who have had Cesareans or have been told to expect one.

My awareness of Cesarean mothers' needs comes from contact with a friend. When her first child was born, she planned to have him at home. Unfortunately, the baby's head was too big to pass through her vaginal canal, and she ended up having an unexpected Cesarean birth. In her case, there was no question that a Cesarean was the only safe way to deliver this child. For some women, however, the issues are not as clear-cut. Having planned for an unmedicated, natural childbirth, they view their Cesarean birth experience as a failure. They are left feeling disappointed, isolated, depressed, and cheated.

It is important that those of you who have experienced Cesareans remember that you are not alone. There are support groups around the country, perhaps even in your city, so you can talk to someone or even attend meetings.

One such group is CARESS, The Cesarean Association for Research Education Support and Satisfaction in Birthing, Inc. This support group, made up of Cesarean couples and medical professionals, provides support and education to expectant parents and the Cesarean family. It also encourages families to take an active role in planning and securing the type of positive, rewarding birth experience desired. Take advantage of the companionship and advice such groups offer. Your worst enemies during the postpartum period are ignorance and isolation. Respect your need to be with other mothers, or simply to talk with another person about your feelings.

The key factor toward a smooth recovery is attitude. Face your feelings. Perhaps you will find it helpful to write them down. Examine the meaning of your birth experience. Undoubtedly you have learned some dramatic lessons. Try to incorporate them into an experience which has culminated in a healthy body. The sooner you accept your feelings about the birth, the more quickly you can move on and let yourself feel a wider range of emotions.

Some of the techniques you learned in the coaching chapter will be very useful now. Focus on the visualizing methods. See yourself doing something you want to be doing. Let that give you a sense of satisfaction and pleasure. See your body healed and moving fully. This can help you to recover more quickly and will create a pleasanter atmosphere while you are healing.

The First Few Days Postpartum

Knowing what to expect the first few days will reduce anxiety and will help make your recovery smoother. You will experience some pain, but this is to be expected. You have had major surgery. You can ask your doctor for pain medication *when* and *if* you need it. And remember to use your breathing techniques (see Chapter 2). They can be extremely helpful in coping with discomfort.

First Day

o You will probably have the Foley catheter removed (unless there is a reason to keep it in longer; ask the nurse about it).
o The first time you get up to go to the bathroom, it may not be easy. Ask for help.

○ Your I.V. might be removed.
○ The hospital might start you on a liquid diet—often gelatin, broth, or tea (you might ask your partner to get you some herb tea instead of black caffeinated tea).
○ You will get to feed the baby. Ask for help if you need it to get into a comfortable position.
○ Remember to keep your visits and calls short. You need your rest! Sleep as much as possible. It will help you heal faster.

Second Day
○ You will begin to feel much stronger, but don't overdo.
○ You might have a fever; however, you still can nurse.
○ Walk frequently but don't get overtired.
○ You may be allowed to shower.

Third Day
○ Move about—walk, walk, walk.
○ Your milk will come in (for some women this happens earlier) so nurse more frequently.
○ Gas pains may occur (see "For Gas," below).
○ Some hospitals let you go home today.

Subsequent Days
○ Move and walk as much as you can, but avoid fatigue.
○ Try to relax. You'll be back on your feet sooner than you think.

For Gas
○ Avoid eating ice, carbonated drinks, lettuce, spicy foods, beans, or caffeinated drinks (coffee, cocoa, or tea).
○ Avoid drinking through a straw.
○ To help expel gas, lie on your left side, then gently knead your abdomen while keeping your knees bent (see Exercise Section). Spreading the buttocks while lying in this position helps pass gas, too.
○ Roll from side to side while you are in bed. The movement helps the gas pass.
○ If you are having trouble moving your bowels, ask the nurse about getting a Harris Flush or a suppository. Keeping your system flushing will help your recovery.

To Minimize Discomfort from Your Incision When You Move

O *Getting out of bed*: Roll over to one side. Sit on the edge of the bed and dangle your feet. Swing your feet back and forth a few times. Don't strain. Brace your buttocks and abdomen as you put the weight on your feet. Lift your upper back and stand tall. Don't lean forward. You can support your incision with your hands for comfort. Now you are ready to begin walking, slowly.

O *Using the toilet*: Ask your nurse to place a wastebasket on its side on the floor in front of the toilet. Put your feet up on it. This can relieve tenderness in your abdomen and help you pass bowel movements. It's almost like squatting on the toilet without the balancing problem.

O If your sanitary belt hurts you or rubs the incision, put a second pad lengthwise under the belt across your pubic area as a cushion against chafing, or use beltless sanitary pads.

O Until the incision is no longer tender, wear cotton nightgowns that do not adhere to your skin.

O Ask for a binder for abdominal support if necessary. It looks like a wide ace bandage.

To Relieve Pain From Spinal Anesthesia

O Force fluids. Drinking really helps.

O Lie flat as much as possible. This can be a wonderful time to engage in your favorite fantasies.

O An abdominal binder may help ease the pain.

To Facilitate Breastfeeding in General

You need special help when you are nursing. Place a pillow between the baby and your incision. This is no time to get an accidental kick. The pillow offers soft protection from unsuspecting feet.

EXERCISES FOR CESAREAN MOMS

The exercises in this section are used by CARESS. They are approved by doctors as safe and will cause no damage to your incision when you do them with awareness and patience. Many of them are variations of exercises in Chapter 2.

Yes, you will have some tenderness for a few days after surgery, so give your abdominal area some support with your hands for a few days. Circulation is the main benefit of these exercises. You want your body to heal as quickly as possible. In fact, you can start right after your operation in the recovery room. If you have been given a general anesthetic, you can start in your hospital bed, with the helpful reminders from your partner.

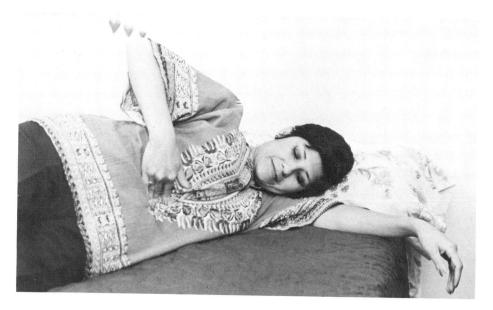

Abdominal Kneading

One of the most painful experiences postpartum is gas. You can alleviate any gas by kneading your abdomen. In fact, you can do it in the recovery room. The anesthetic, unless you have had a general, can help you to touch your abdomen with less fear of pain.

Place your hand 4 inches *above* your incision. If you want, you can put your other hand over your incision to support it or make contact with it. Knead on your abdomen (a bit below your bustline) as if kneading dough. Let your fingers move like caterpillars across your abdomen, vertically and horizontally. This will help your intestines move the gas through. Be sure *not* to knead your uterus. By massaging your abdomen as often as you can after surgery, you can avoid a lot of discomfort.

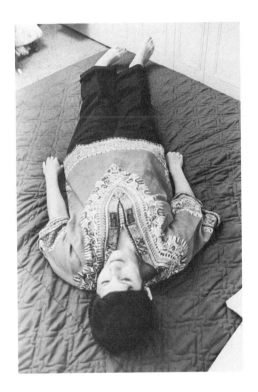

Ankle Works

This exercise helps to reduce swelling and minimize varicose veins. It also helps to improve your foot and leg circulation. Simply stretch your feet in all directions, forward and back, side to side. Then circle your foot in one direction, then the opposite direction. You can do this lying down or sitting in a chair, but don't try to do it while you are walking. This is a wonderful exercise to do when you want to pass the time more quickly in recovery.

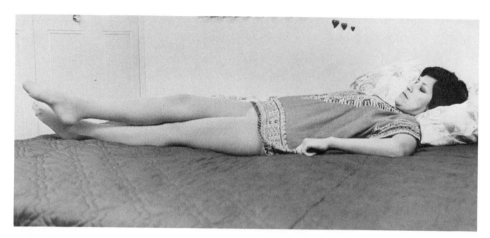

Leg Toner

For a short while you will not be as active as you are used to being, so you will need exercises to increase circulation to your legs. They will help the circulation all the way up to your buttocks.

Lie on your back, legs straight in front. Cross your ankles. Press your legs together. Tense your knees, then your thigh muscles, and finally squeeze your buttocks together. Hold for a few seconds and relax.

Let the tensing be progressive: start low and work your way up to your buttocks gradually. Be sure to breathe while you do this.

Kegel

Yes, even as a Cesarean mother you need to retone your vaginal canal. The added weight of your baby during pregnancy affected the tone of the vaginal muscles. The *Kegels* will improve circulation and assist in the healing process.

As you tighten slowly, focus on the tensing part, not the relaxing part. Contract the muscle for five counts and relax for four counts.

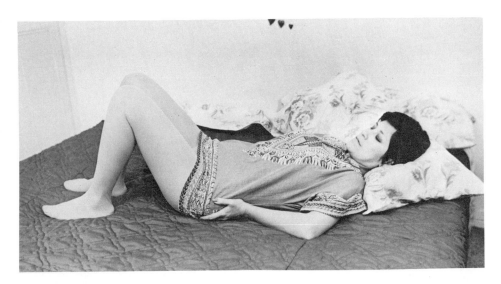

Pelvic Rocks

Your main aim here is to stimulate sluggish intestinal activity, not to strengthen your muscles. Rock *gently*, focusing your attention on your torso.

Lie on your back and bend your knees. Press the small of your back into the bed or floor. Arch it off the bed, pressing and arching, and continue rocking your pelvis gently.

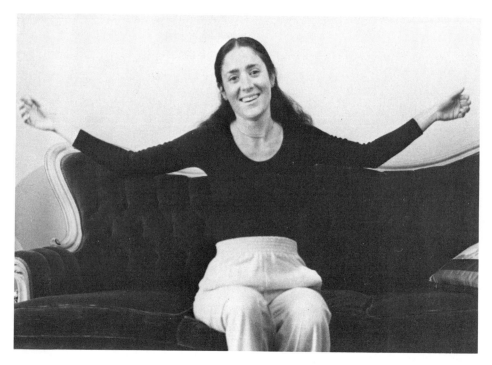

Milkmaid

Now that you are nursing, this exercise helps relax the muscles in your chest, which in turn helps your milk come in more easily. These movements will be the same as when you were pregnant (see Chapter 2), only much easier and slower. For a variation, you can put your hands on your shoulders and rotate your shoulders in both directions. Relax your hands down and stretch your arms to the back, and then swing the arms forward gently.

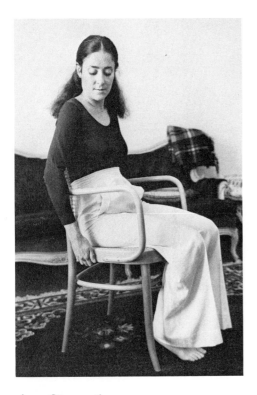

Arm Strengthener

You will be depending on your arms now more than before. It's a good idea to strengthen them for holding the baby and for supporting your body when you sit up.

Sit on a chair. Grasp the seat tightly, elbows bent. Try to pull the bottom of the chair up toward you. Then push the bottom away. For each action, count one through five. Alternate pulling and pushing. Relax in between each full cycle.

Another variation is using the hospital bed rails. Lie down on your back in bed. Grasp the hand rails firmly. Pull on them to activate the muscles in your arms without lifting your body. See if you can feel it in your upper arms. Relax and try pushing away from the rails. Remember to breathe.

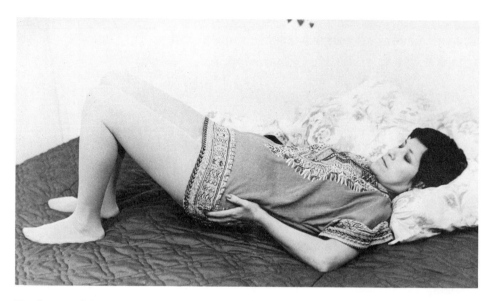

Bridge and Twist

This should not be done until the sixth week after your birth. A member of CARESS tells me that some women say they experience some discomfort when they do this. You do want to improve your abdominal circulation, but not strain or hurt yourself. So be gentle when you do this exercise. Twist your hips right and left only as far as you feel comfortable. Relax with the movement. Lie flat on the bed, and then lift your buttocks off the bed. Hold this elevated position and twist your hips to the right and then to the left. Lower your buttocks back to the bed. Relax.

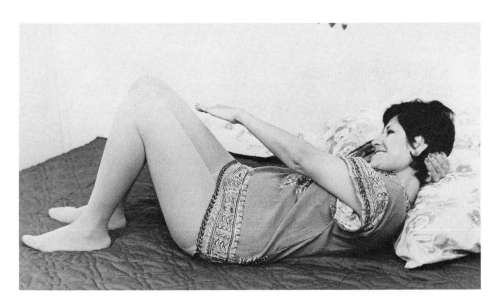

Tummy Toner

This exercise should also be done at six weeks. You can retone your abdominal muscles and also stretch the back of your neck when you tuck your chin down. Lie on your back with the back of the bed raised or several pillows under your head and shoulders. Exhale and tuck your chin down. Reach forward toward your knees with your hands. Hold for a moment. Inhale as you lower your head. Return your shoulders to the bed. Relax and repeat.

For additional comfort, you might want to support the incision with one hand while you reach with the other.

If you feel any strain with the exercise, place one hand behind your neck and reach for your knees with your head and free arm. See if that helps you do the movement with less stress.

As you exercise, have patience with yourself. You are recovering from surgery. Acknowledge your limitations and make the best of them. You will help yourself by practicing these gentle movements and by talking with other mothers.

193

Going Home

Going home from the hospital is a big event for you and your new family. You will want help at first. Arrange for a friend, relative, or another pregnant woman who would love the experience of being near a newborn, to lend a hand. Your main job is to rest and recover. Remember that you have just had a baby plus abdominal surgery. You have two people to take care of—a new little person and yourself. Let someone else help with the housework, laundry, marketing, and cooking.

Be sure to set aside time to talk about your reaction to the birth. Respect and acknowledge your feelings, whatever they are. Often the father feels a mixture of emotions. If he was prepared to see the birth and was asked to leave the delivery room, he might have some feelings of disappointment. You may have some negative feelings, too. Try not to take them out on each other. Focus instead on the joy of seeing your new baby, the relief that it's all over, and the love you feel toward your new family.

Remember that support groups can be very helpful now; you can either attend meetings or get help over the phone. Two months after the birth you can begin the postpartum exercises suggested in the first half of this chapter. Don't rush. Get back into your schedule slowly. Patience now will pay off later.

7. New to the world: exercising the baby

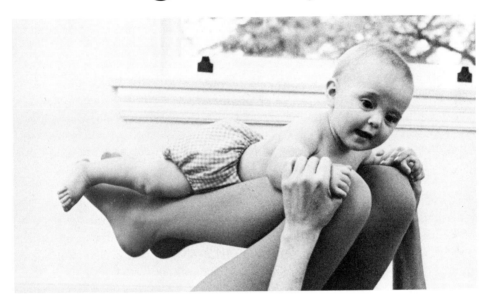

Newborns appear so fragile. In fact, they are quite sturdy. Being born is hard work. First our heads are molded so they are able to pass through the pelvis; we are abruptly expelled from our mothers' bodies; we must experience that first breath on our own. Even the gentlest of births is labor, both for mother and for baby.

Try to visualize your baby's environment for the last nine months. Floating and bobbing in water provides a very different kind of support system than air. What was initially a spacious palace has gradually grown more and more cramped, causing the limbs to flex and curl into the body. Think what it must be like to be suddenly thrust into the air.

Don't expect your newborn to look like the infants in baby food ads. The head may be temporarily elongated from the birth process, during which the skull bones overlap to allow the head to pass through the pelvis. These bones will fuse together gradually as the baby matures. If forceps were used in the birth, you may notice bruises on the head. Such birthmarks often go away within a year. Sometimes the ears and nose are flattened or distorted temporarily because of the way the baby was positioned in the uterus, or as a result of the trip down the birth canal. If silver nitrate was used, the eyes may be puffy for a day or two after the birth.

If your baby is under 7 pounds, the skin may appear wrinkled or loose for the first few weeks. But infants fill in quickly and from day one uphold their reputation for having the softest skin in the world. The vernix, or white coating which covers them at birth, offers protection before they are born.

Newborns often have a yellowish appearance. This is due to a break-down of red blood cells with which the baby is born. It is called *physiologic jaundice* and often is "relieved" by placing the baby in direct sunlight or under lights. If there is a problem, your doctor will advise you. When Anna was a day old she was a bit yellow, so we went out in the back yard for half an hour every day. The condition cleared up quickly, with no problems. Sometimes there is fine hair like peach fuzz on the body. This is called *lanugo* and it soon disappears.

Dark-bluish areas are sometimes seen on the buttocks or lower back, or on nonwhite babies. They are called *Mongolian spots* and will soon fade. The small white spots on the nose and forehead are called *millia*. They, too, go away by themselves. Another phenomenon is the swelling of genitals of both sexes. This is due to the increased amount of hormones in the mother at birth. Such hormones can also affect the breasts of the newborn, making them swell or secrete a fluid. Baby girls may have slight "menstrual" bleeding for the same reason. There is no cause for alarm; the symptoms go away without treatment.

GETTING TO KNOW YOUR NEWBORN

Infants have a lot of adjusting to do. So do first-time parents. An awareness of what to expect will make those first days easier for all concerned. Here are some things to watch for:

Your baby may be easily chilled, with feet that are bluish or cold. Infants should be kept warm but not overdressed. They can't sweat yet.

Newborns are likely to hiccup frequently, especially while nursing. I used to think Anna was getting drunk on my milk. Her so-called hiccups were actually normal spasms from her developing diaphragm. I found gentle burping and holding were the best remedies.

Infants often lose weight the first few days. Since they are born with extra stores of fluid in their bodies, they are prepared for this. For the first few days the baby may not seem hungry. There is no cause to worry. The appetite soon picks up. You will be nursing more often once the newborn adjusts to being here. Don't be alarmed if the baby develops a sucking blister on the lip. This is normal.

Nursing is an adjustment for both Mom and the baby. You, as mother, will need to keep your nutrition well balanced. You will find that eating grains such as rice, millet, wheatberries, and alfalfa sprouts increases milk production. Blessed thistle is a wonderful tea to drink to relax you and help milk production. When you begin nursing, find yourself a comfortable nursing bra. I lived in mine for the first three months. I needed the support.

Don't be surprised if you get a *let-down reflex*. This is the term which describes leakage from one breast while the baby nurses the other. It can occur if you simply *think* about nursing. Breast pads can be helpful here to keep from soaking your tops. Make sure the pads allow your nipples to "breathe." Beware of pads backed by plastic coatings. They can cause sore nipples. And remember, a good book can help make nursing a success. Karen Pryor's book, *Nursing Your Baby*, was especially useful to me. The La Leche League is also there to give support and advice. Consult your local group. The baby will let you know when he or she is hungry. One lesson I learned was to feed first, diaper next. They don't care if they're wet, but hunger is a crisis to be solved immediately.

The first bowel movement the baby will have is called *meconium*. It is dark and tarrish looking. Should this first stool stick to your baby's skin, use oil to loosen it gently. In the beginning, don't be alarmed if the stools are a greenish color; this is often an indication that the liver is cleaning house. Later, stools will have a light yellowish brown color. It is normal for a breastfed baby to have loose stools, sometimes one after each feeding, sometimes one every two days! There is a wide range of what is considered normal frequency.

Newborns have a complex set of reflexes. Their arms or legs jerk suddenly when they are startled. This is known as the *Moro reflex*. Babies can lift and turn their heads by themselves. Anna lifted her head in the first week and then stopped for three months! In the first week there is a stepping reflex. The baby looks as if he or she is walking on a tightrope, one foot carefully placed before the other. Newborns are able to suck on nearly anything presented to them. Some babies have a greater need to suck than others. They also have a grasping reflex. Watch out, their grip is strong! They also yawn, sneeze, blink, stretch, and look around.

One word here about mobiles. Most mobiles are made to be looked at from the side. Get underneath them and see what the baby will be looking up at. You might want to rearrange the way the objects are hung, or restring them so that the baby will see the sides and not the bottom.

Infants have excellent hearing. They began listening to your body sounds before they were born. The sounds of blood pulsing, food digesting, kidneys filtering, belching, talking, and breathing are all familiar to your newborn. Yet once babies emerge into the world, many new parents protect their infants from noise. True, you don't want horns honking in their ears, but you don't have to tiptoe around your house while the baby is sleeping either. Most newborns quickly get used to normal noises. In fact I think some babies miss the sounds they were exposed to before birth, just as they may miss the constant motion—after all, they *do* like to be rocked.

It is helpful for new parents to remember that babies are resilient. They can tolerate those first mistakes we often make. I'll never forget the first time I stuck Anna with a diaper pin. She howled, of course, and I felt paralyzed by guilt. But once I realized that what she needed was a fresh diaper and a cuddle rather than my remorse, we went right on with our day as if nothing had happened. It was a lesson I never forgot.

MOVING WITH YOUR BABY

Moving with your baby for the first few months consists largely of holding, hugging, rocking, and cradling. The most important thing to remember is to move the baby slowly and gently, supporting the head with the hand under the upper neck and the head, keeping the head, neck and chest in much the same plane, until the neck muscles are well developed. All of the baby's limbs have been flexed, with their arms pulled in, legs bent, neck forward. Open and stretch all the limbs slowly. Open and close their joints—the shoulders, elbows, wrists, hip sockets, knees, and feet. This can be done right from the start if the mother feels up to it and the sluggishness of the baby has disappeared. The ideal time is when the baby is being sponge-bathed, if the cord hasn't fallen off. Feel when they don't want to stretch. Songs or varying rhythms can help you both relax. Sometimes you have to wait for their mood to coincide with yours, before they are willing to open and stretch. I found the bathtub a good place to relax and stretch with my daughter after the umbilical cord had fallen off (it takes from one to two weeks). She was more relaxed and we were able to explore movement possibilities in a fluid environment. I would take her into the tub with me and help her float. She enjoyed it a lot. Perhaps it reminded her of the womb.

Never force babies to go beyond their limits. Let them tell you what they can do. *Listen, watch, and learn from their reactions.* (Never lift newborns up by the hands only. You might dislocate the shoulders if you jerk them up too quickly or try to carry them around that way.)

By the time your baby is almost two months old you will be able to start a more extensive exercise program. The exercises in this chapter are divided into two sections: those for the very beginner, and those for older babies. I have suggested ages at which to start the advanced exercises, but use your own judgment. If your baby appears able to do them sooner, fine. If not, be patient. The right time will come. Remember, your baby will set his or her own pace. These exercises are designed to be fun for you both. They are not a means of comparison or competition between one baby and another.

The surface you choose to exercise on needs to be firm yet cushioned— a wooden floor or carpeted floor can be padded with a baby blanket, a soft towel, or an exercise mat. You could also move the baby on a firm bed. Try to exercise the same time each day. At first, establishing a routine can be difficult, but after the first three months you and the baby should be able to arrive at a suitable mutual time. A baby's schedule is more flexible than you might think. You're not the only one who should have to adjust.

Anna and I exercised *every* day from her third month until her first birthday. She would almost remind me if I forgot. That first year of exercising gave her a good sense of her body. She loves to move and dance even now. We still "exercise" together but now it is more like playing and dancing than following a strict routine.

Of course children learn how to sit up, crawl, and walk even if we never touch them, but it is a joy to be integrally involved in moving with them. I can see that Anna has a confidence in the way she moves that many children her age who have not had such movement experiences lack.

As you exercise with your baby, don't hesitate to improvise. If you aren't sure the baby can do something, try it slowly. The baby will let you know how she or he feels about what you are doing. Together you can create your own dance—a baby dance.

WAYS TO HOLD THE BABY

FOOTBALL HOLD: Place one hand under the belly, grasping firmly.
DOUBLE HAND SWING: With baby facing forward, clasp hands, put baby in between, and relax arms.
OVER THE SHOULDER: Remember to switch sides from time to time.
HIPPY PARENT: Holding the baby on one hip, then the other.
THE CRADLE: Cradle the baby in both arms.

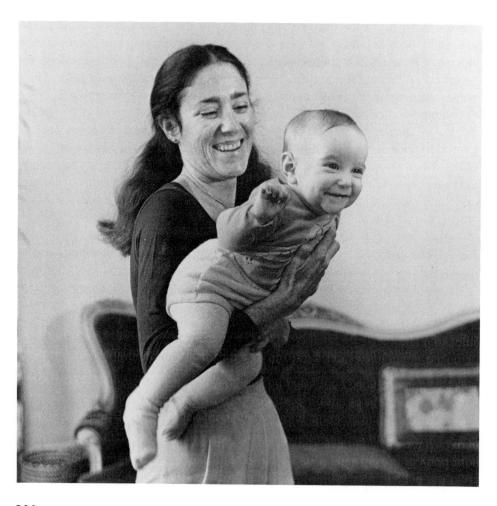

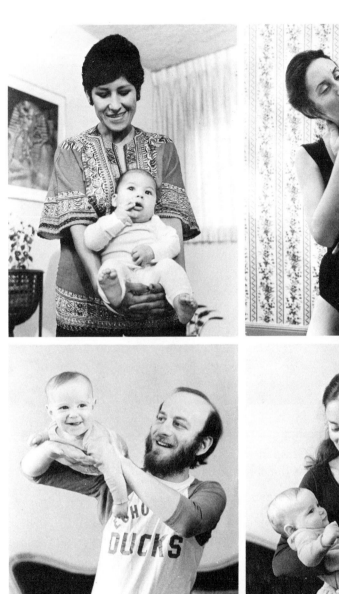

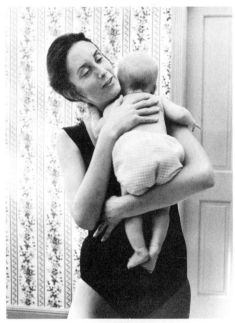

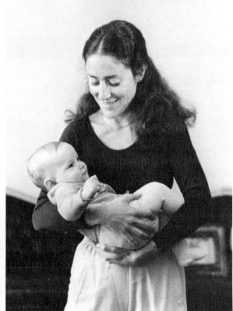

EXERCISES FOR BABY

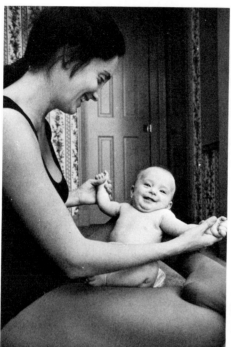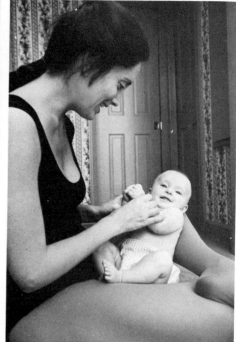

Hug Me Tight

Place your baby on his back. Grasp his wrists and gently stretch his arms out to the sides. Now fold the arms across the chest, as if your baby is hugging himself.

Repeat the cycle, alternating the arm you fold in first.

After being cramped for months, a baby's arms need to be opened and stretched, especially at the shoulder joints. This exercise also helps your baby breathe more fully.

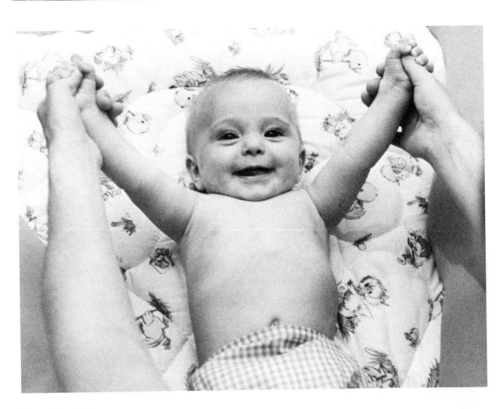

The Stretch

Place your baby on her back. Hold onto one wrist and gently raise the arm over the head. Alternate arms.

Next, hold onto both wrists and raise both arms together, gently and slowly. Lower both arms.

Repeat, varying the rhythm.

By encouraging your baby to move fully, you foster a sense of confidence in the environment. You may sense your baby's resistance to being stretched, but if you go slowly and gently, eventually her arms will open all the way.

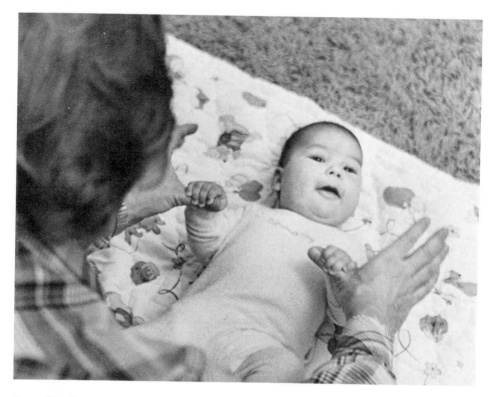

Arm Circles

Place your baby on his back and grasp one wrist. Let the other arm relax. Gently draw circles in front, to the side, and overhead with the arm you are holding. Reverse the direction of the circles. Repeat with other arm. Then gently circle both arms together.

This exercise explores and expands the range of movement possible in each shoulder socket.

Each of the arm exercises helps your baby explore a specific range of movement. You can add to the fun by playing your favorite music. I found singing along with the record helped me and Anna relax and "dance" through the movements. She didn't seem to care if my voice was off key, or if I made up new words. Improvising was fun.

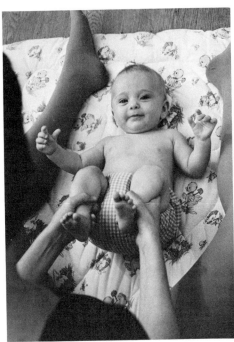 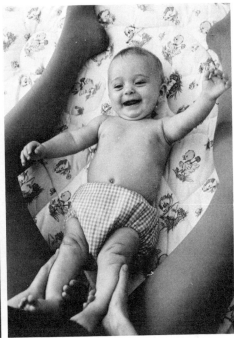

Kick-a-Poo Kid

Place your baby on her back. Grasp both legs behind the knee. Bend one knee and gently pull to stretch and straighten it. Alternate sides.

Let the baby start to kick with some resistance from you.

Try different rhythms.

Kicking builds leg muscles.

Learning to walk takes most babies nine to fourteen months. If they exercise their legs early, they are helped to build muscles while they are not bearing weight.

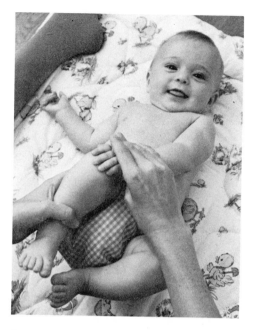

Bring 'Em Together

Place your baby on his back. Take hold of the right wrist and the back of the right knee. Bring the hand and knee together slowly, then gently pull down to stretch them long. The arm should stretch overhead, the leg should be stretched out fully on the floor. Repeat on the other side.

Next, bring the right hand and the left knee together, and stretch them long in the same manner. Repeat with the left hand and the right knee.

This is a great warm-up exercise. It also stimulates the intestines and helps relieve gas pains. It facilitates coordination in the hip and shoulder sockets, as well as acquainting your baby with right and left side movement.

I suggest you try *Bring 'Em Together* before you do *Cross Crawling*. It serves as a warm-up. All of this movement is leading up to what happens when a baby crawls.

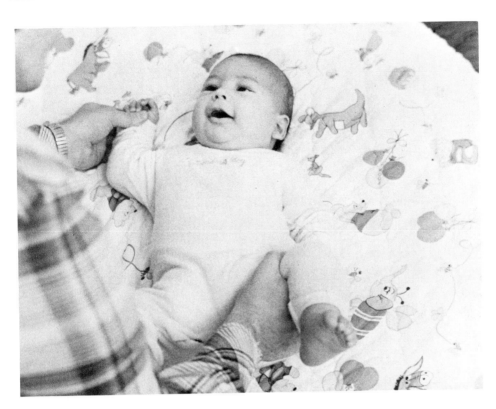

Cross Crawling

Place your baby on her back. Take hold of the right arm and the back of the left knee. Simultaneously raise the right arm over the head and the left knee toward the abdomen. Return the arm and leg to the floor. Reverse the exercise: raise both the left arm and right knee and lower them slowly to the floor.

This movement pattern imitates the beginning movements of crawling. It also stimulates the arm and leg muscles to stretch and move together. Also, stretching the thigh toward the abdomen helps to massage the baby's intestines. If your baby has gas or discomfort, this exercise can help relieve it.

At first both you and your baby might feel a little awkward with this coordination pattern. Remember, go slowly. If you do this exercise consistently, your baby will learn and enjoy the movement with you.

Cross Crawling is also used for older children who have learning disabilities because it helps balance the right and left centers of the brain.

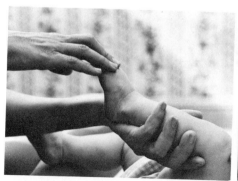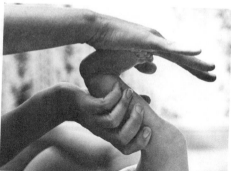

A-Boot-a-Stretch

Place your baby on his back. Take hold of one leg. With your other hand gently press his foot forward and back (pointing and flexing). Repeat on the other side.

Babies are born with their feet curved. This exercise helps to stretch their shin and calf muscles, as well as strengthening the feet.

As your baby gets older, let him push your hand with his foot while you give him gentle resistance.

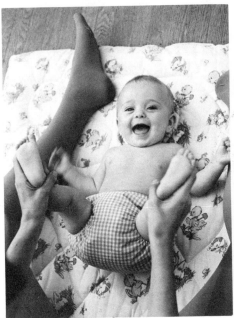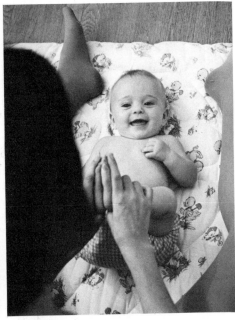

Feet Clappers

Place your baby on her back. Hold onto both ankles. Bring the soles of the feet together, in a clapping motion. Then gently stretch (turn) the balls of the feet away from each other. Alternate clapping and stretching.

Look at your baby's feet. Do they tend to turn in one direction or another? Most babies' feet sickle in so that the foot looks like a comma. This exercise helps strengthen the muscles on both sides of your baby's lower legs.

Feet Clappers is especially helpful for babies who have been put in corrective shoes. It helps to straighten out the muscles that cause the foot to curve in or out.

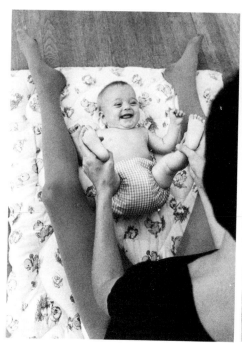
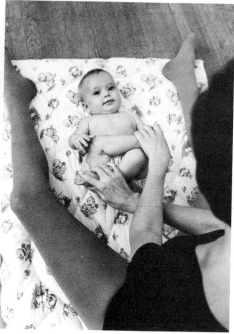

Crisscross—Yogi Stretch

Place your baby on his back. Grasp both feet. Cross the legs by gently pulling the right foot toward the left and the left foot toward the right.

Next, slowly raise the crossed legs toward the tummy. As you lower the legs to the floor, open them slowly and stretch them out long on the floor. Repeat the whole sequence with the opposite leg on top.

This exercise is wonderful for opening and stretching the hip sockets while increasing the range of movement in the legs. But proceed gently. Listen and look for any sign of discomfort from your baby. If there is discomfort, stop. Do the movement smaller, go slower, or wait and do it at a later time.

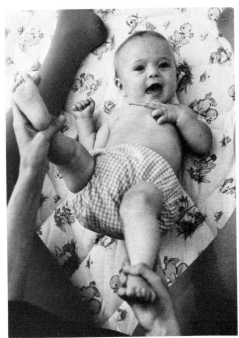 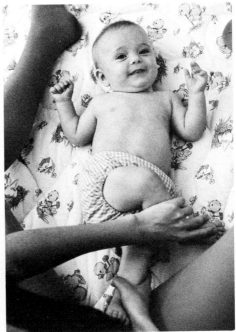

Toe Tapping

Place your baby on her back. Grasp the right foot. Tap it on the baby's left thigh and then tap it on the floor outside of the left leg. Return both buttocks to the floor, and stretch the leg out straight on the floor. Repeat with the left foot.

This series of exercises is geared to make the baby more aware of movement in the thigh and hip sockets. It increases the range of movement while strengthening the muscles in the legs and thighs.

I used to sing a song to Anna while doing this exercise. She came to associate the song with the movement and almost seemed to hum along with me.

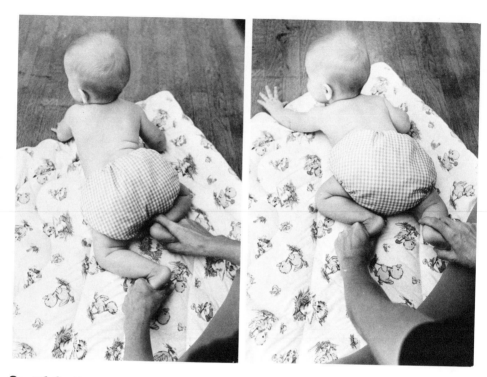

Scuttlebutt

Place your baby on his stomach. Bend both knees and tuck them under the body. Press your palms against the feet and let your baby push forward. Repeat by again tucking the feet up in back of the body. Watch the baby scoot forward.

This exercise strengthens the leg muscles your baby will use for crawling. I see babies experience such joy at being able to "move" for themselves. Often when babies start to crawl, the movement is backward no matter how hard they try to move ahead. I remember how Anna used to crawl toward something and end up further away than when she started. Doing this exercise relieved some of her frustration.

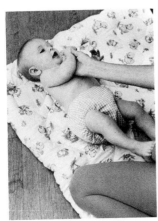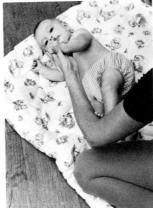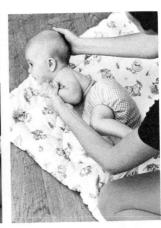

Roll Me Over

Place your baby on her back. Bend her right knee and grasp her right wrist. Slowly roll her over onto her tummy. Straighten her left arm.

To roll the baby over onto her back, put one hand behind her head. Hold onto her right shoulder while you gently roll her over onto her back. Repeat, rolling to the other side.

Learning to roll over is a major achievement for babies. This exercise allows you to help. However, even before your baby can roll over by herself, be sure to watch where you put her down. If she is on a bed, surround her with pillows which will act as a barrier.

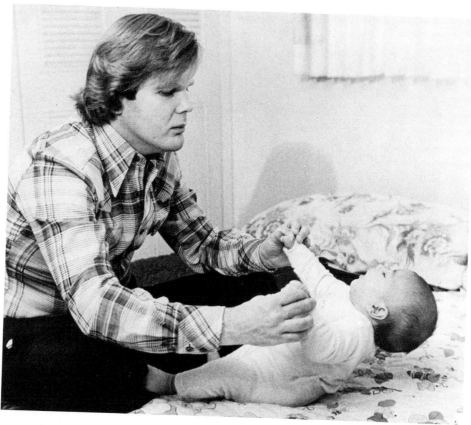

*Hold Tight*_____

Place your baby on his back. Let the baby put both his hands around one of yours, use your other hand to support the head and neck. Raise the baby slowly into a sitting position. Slowly lower the baby back onto the blanket.

This exercise is especially useful for strengthening the abdominal and arm muscles as well as giving the grasping muscles in the hands a good workout. In the beginning you will need a helping hand to support your baby's head. You know what is behind his head, but he doesn't. It can be scary at first, so be patient. Your baby's trust in you will grow each day.

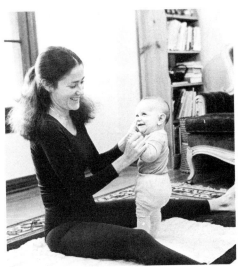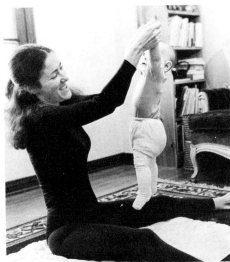

Up, Up and Away

When your baby is able to stand on her own, let her hold onto your hands. Give a gentle tug to feel some resistance. Slowly lift the baby. When your baby is strong enough, you can continue to lift her until she is off the ground entirely.

This is a more advanced exercise and works to strengthen hands, arms, shoulders, and abdominal muscles.

A variation of this exercise is to hold a tempting object in front of the baby and let her pull herself up to sitting and then standing, as far as possible. As your child learns to crawl and maneuver around the house, she will start to pull herself up on everything. This is practice for just that kind of activity, except now *you* are around to help and play.

One of the first ways your baby will begin to connect with her world is through her mouth and hands. Babies are born with a grasping reflex. As they grow older, you can stimulate that reflex by giving them something to hold on to. They probably won't start reaching by themselves until they are four or five months old. My daughter used to love this exercise. Not only did she want to sit—she wanted to stand, for most of the day. We had a lot of fun watching the joy in her face when she could stand on her feet. Her grip became extremely strong. She now can hang from a bar all by herself. She trusts her hands because she knows they have the strength to hold her.

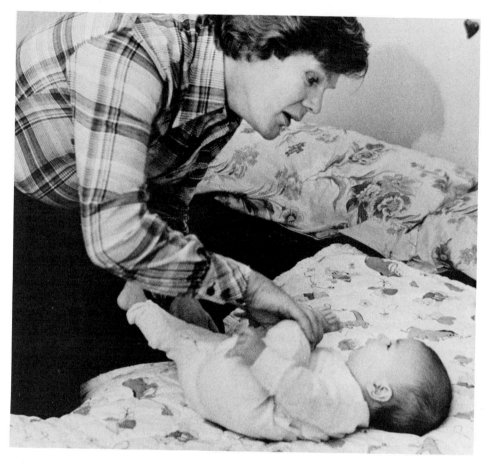

Shoulder Tapping

Place your baby on his back. Grasp his right foot. Slowly stretch the foot and leg toward the left shoulder. Return the foot to the floor. Repeat, stretching the left foot toward the right shoulder.

This exercise stretches the lower back, stretches the back of the thigh, and opens up movement in the hip socket. It is also great for massaging the intestines. This is another excellent exercise for babies with gas or blocked bowels.

When I first did this with Anna, her hips were too tight for her foot to reach her shoulder. However, after doing it for a few weeks, she loosened up enough to reach it.

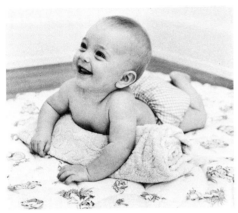 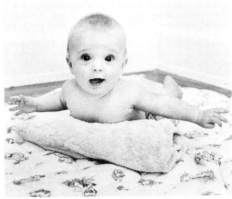

Back Arch

Place your baby on his stomach. Roll a bath towel and place it under the baby's chest. Let him push up with his arms.

The towel helps the baby arch his back. This exercise helps the muscles in the small of the back to grow stronger.

Back arching is a preliminary step in helping your baby learn how to sit up, which requires use of the muscles in both the abdomen and the back. Until sitting up is possible, at least he can get his nose off the floor. I used to watch Anna feel so frustrated because she wanted to see more than the floor. With the towel under her chest she could look around the room. I decided to put some bright pictures at her eye level so she would have something more interesting to look at than walls or the underside of tables.

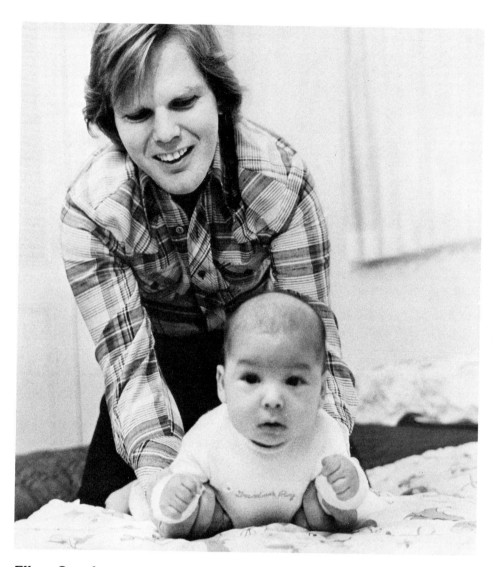

Elbow Stand

Place the baby on his stomach. Prop both elbows under his body. Watch and see how long the baby can comfortably support himself on his elbows.

This exercise helps to build the muscles in the shoulder girdle and middle back. It also gives a baby the chance to use his arms for support before he learns to pull himself across the floor.

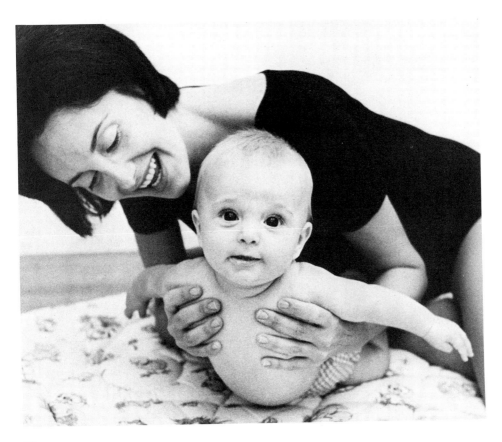

Flying

Place your baby on her stomach. Grasp both upper arms and gently stretch the arms out to the sides as you lift and arch the baby's back. Slowly return the chest to the floor.

Before your baby can sit up, there are several sets of muscles that must develop: the head and neck muscles, the abdominal muscles, and the back muscles. This exercise focuses on developing the back muscles.

Pay special attention to how your baby lifts up her body. If you feel any tension or resistance to arching, stop. Ease into this exercise slowly and gently. Here again, let your baby set the pace.

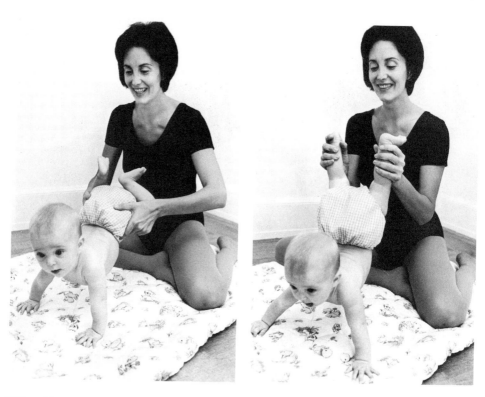

Wheelbarrow

Place your baby on his stomach. Grasp both hips and slowly lift the hips off the ground. Let your baby support himself on his hands. Eventually his arms will be strong enough to hold up his body. Later, your baby may be able to "walk" forward on his hands!

This is a wonderful exercise for strengthening the muscles in the arms and shoulders.

If you detect any strain as you enjoy this exercise with your baby, stop. Don't try to push your baby. His muscles will develop at their own pace. There is no rush to have him walking around on his hands.

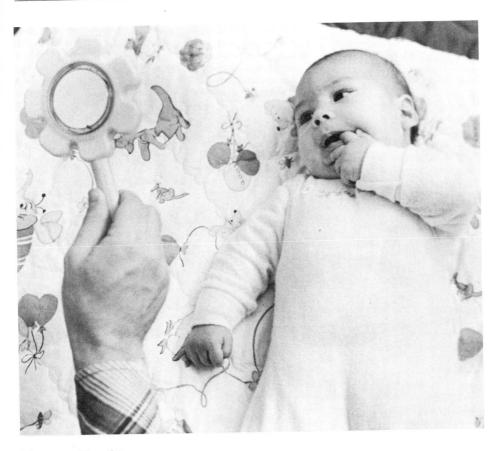

Keep on Tracking

Place your baby on his back. Hold a brightly colored noise-making object, such as a rattle, directly over the baby's head. Make a noise until the baby makes eye contact with the object. Slowly move the object to the right and the left. Watch and see if your baby's eyes follow the object. Eventually the baby will reach for the object.

Visual stimulation and movement all help the baby's ability to see and focus. This exercise helps strengthen the eye and tracking muscles.

Use your imagination in choosing objects for this exercise. Vary colors, shapes, sizes, textures. Anna especially liked shiny things from our kitchen. You don't have to go out and buy new things. Often something in the house that you are used to looking at is fascinating and novel to your baby.

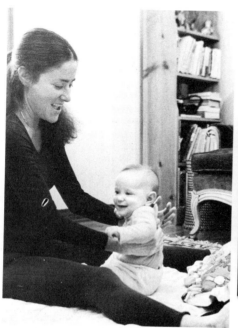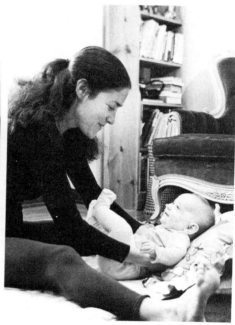

Kaboom

Put a large, soft pillow on the floor. Place your baby on her back with the head and back supported by the pillow. The first time you do this exercise, place one hand behind the baby's head. Sit the baby up and let her "fall" gently back toward the pillow. As your baby gets used to falling, you no longer need to support her head.

This is one of the best exercises I know to help babies learn how to fall without fear. In the process of learning how to crawl and walk, they are constantly pulling themselves up, crawling off things, or falling. Watching older babies learn how to walk is a constant process of up and "kaboom" down on their bottoms.

Much of the fear comes from not being relaxed about falling. I practiced this exercise with Anna often and now she rarely cries when she falls down. She picks herself up and continues to move where she left off. I also think that many babies cry when they fall because of the way grownups react to it. If you rush right over and get excited or nervous, the child learns this is something wrong or bad, something to react to with fear and tears. Of course, attention is necessary if there is a problem or injury that needs loving care, but most falls are dry runs for learning how to walk.

8. Exercises for the new family

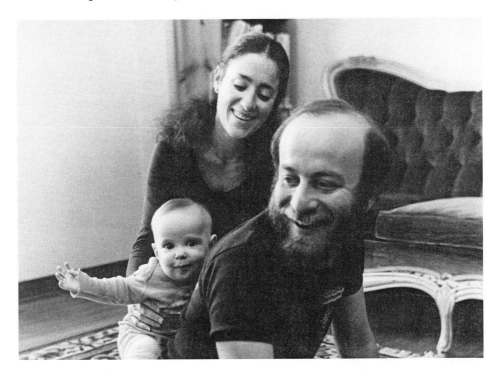

When I became pregnant, some of my friends said, "Just wait and see. Once you have a child you'll have to slow down and do less." Nothing could have been further from the truth. Just as I have adapted to my daughter's needs, she has adapted to mine.

When I was ready to go back to teaching childbirth classes, she came along with me. She fit right in. My students loved having the opportunity to hold a baby, see her get changed and nursed, and watch her learn how to crawl, walk, and talk. I used a front pack to carry Anna for the first five months. She loved going about with me, seeing the world from my shoulder height. I believe it is important for all new parents to realize that young babies are flexible—that they delight in new people and places, that early exposure paves the way for a more sociable, adaptable adulthood.

As a dancer, I was impatient to begin moving as soon after childbirth as possible. Why not use this precious time at home with my newborn, I thought, to develop a system of movements Anna and I could do together that would keep us *both* in shape? As I experimented with Anna in my arms, I came to feel more and more that she was an extension of my body. This made me feel freer to move, to use my feet and legs, to develop the exercises that follow.

One day at a postnatal exercise class I was teaching, a father appeared. He wanted to learn how to move and exercise with his baby. Anna and the other babies in the class seemed to enjoy moving with him. They beamed—he beamed back. It made me start thinking about fathers' roles in parenting. They often feel left out, at a loss as to how to nurture their child. Exercise is a fine solution; it offers a source of closeness which is both pleasurable and educational. After all, babies love to be held.

So, Dad, the following exercises are for you as well as Mom. But one note of caution to fathers. Please don't push your babies to achieve. They will learn at their own pace. Remember, *never* force any movement on a baby. Another word of warning: Don't toss a baby under a year old too violently or too high in the air. The landing is often jarring for his insides. Be gentle. You will have plenty of time to toss and tumble later.

The exercises that follow can also be a way for *both* parents to move with the baby. Set aside time to play together as a new family. If you have other children, they can join in and add to the fun. Use music, sing, or play percussion instruments for accompaniment. There is a wealth of amusement and joy to be found from moving, dancing, being physical *together*.

A final word. We are living in a different age than our parents. I think the most valuable thing we can impart to our children in this rapidly changing world is a sense of faith in themselves as people, as individuals. My moving and exercising with Anna has given her confidence in her body and how it works. She moves with grace and ease. You can give this gift to *your* child, a gift of lifelong value.

As you move through the following exercises, start out slowly and gradually build. If you don't feel like doing a whole set, pick out whatever feels right. As you move together, hug the child in your arms and love her for who she is. This will help her grow to her full potential, ready to interact with her world.

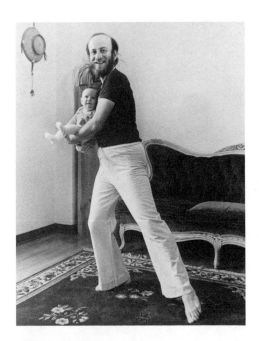

Torso Twister

Stand with your feet parallel, approximately shoulder-width apart. Hold the baby close to your chest. Let your eyes, head, shoulders, ribs, and waist twist to the right, then the left. Keep your hips facing forward for the first few times.

Then, as you twist to the right, let your left heel come off the ground. Rotate back to center. Repeat on other side, and continue to alternate. Slow down gradually.

There is something very relaxing about the swinging motion. Gentle twisting and rocking eases the tension we build up daily. It does wonders to quiet a fretful baby.

To loosen your torso further, try this variation. Twist to the right and notice the farthest point you can see as you turn. Do this a few times to "mark" visually how far you can see. Now, return to the center. Twist again, but this time turn your head in the opposite direction from your shoulders (if you are twisting to the right, turn your head to the left). Repeat for a few twists, returning to a forward position each time. Stop. Now go back to rotating your shoulders and head together. Notice how far you can see now. It will probably be further than before. Sometimes by creating a counter movement we can loosen up muscle groups far faster than by repeating the same pattern over and over again.

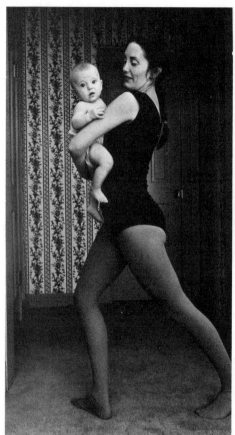 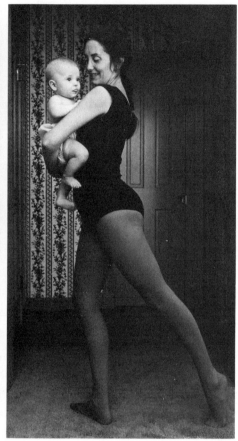

Calf Stretcher

Stand with your feet together, toes turned out slightly. Hold your baby close to you, centered against your body. Step straight back with one foot. Keep your weight on your front foot. Bend your front knee.

Inhale and gently stretch your back heel toward the floor. Exhale and swing your back leg forward. Raise the thigh toward your chest. Inhale and lower your foot to the floor.

Repeat. Take your other leg back, stretch, and kick.

226

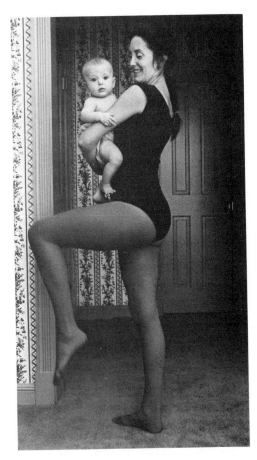

To counteract our wearing high-heeled shoes and our neglecting to lead with our heels when we walk, our calves need stretching every day. Holding the baby gives your arms something to do, and gives the baby a ride.

Balance becomes an interesting problem for you when you swing your back leg forward. Let your supporting leg "grow roots" and become planted into the floor. Balance comes from letting our weight connect us to the ground.

227

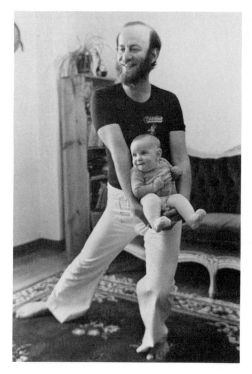

Thigh Toner

Stand with your feet shoulder-width apart, slightly turned out, toes pointing toward the sides. Hold your baby close to you, centered against your chest.

Bend your knees and sway from side to side. Don't forget to breathe. Lower your body, keeping your torso as straight as possible. Bend your knees more. Sway toward your right leg. Press down into the ball of your right foot, exhale and push off. Feel the moment of suspension as your right foot leaves the ground.

Inhale and lightly "fall" back onto your right foot. Repeat five times. Reverse sides.

This exercise helped me regain strength and tone in my thighs and ankle muscles after giving birth. If you don't feel this exercise in your thighs, bend your knees further. Avoid leaning forward from the hips. When you lean forward, you are working another set of muscles. Later you can try both variations. Notice what each feels like to you. What muscles are you using with each position? Decide which muscles need the most attention.

228

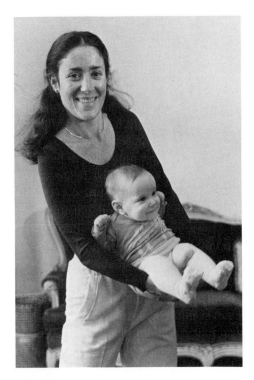

Swingin' Baby

Hold the baby in the crook of your right arm. Swing the baby diagonally across your body to the left side. Swing back to your right side. Continue swinging back and forth for a few minutes. Repeat on the other side.

You will be swinging, holding, and carrying your baby for a long time. You'll want your arm muscles to be strong. Start this exercise early while your baby is still light. This way you can build your arm and shoulder muscles as he puts on weight.

I enjoyed doing this exercise in front of a mirror or facing another person. Anna enjoyed it too.

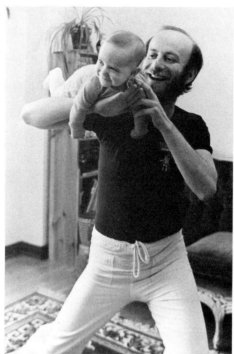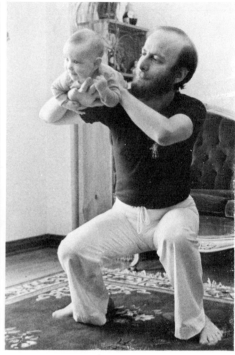

Flying Machine

Stand. Gently raise your arm up level with your shoulder. Rest the baby on top of your shoulder and arm. Use your other hand to steady the baby.

Move about the room, varying your rhythm, speed, and arm height. Lift and straighten your elbow slowly and gently. Repeat with the other arm.

Most people have excess flab on their underarms. This exercise directly works on toning that flab back into firm muscle. Experiment with different kinds of music and rhythms. I loved to hold Anna and dance toward a mirror, then walk backwards slowly. Anna would laugh and smile at her reflection.

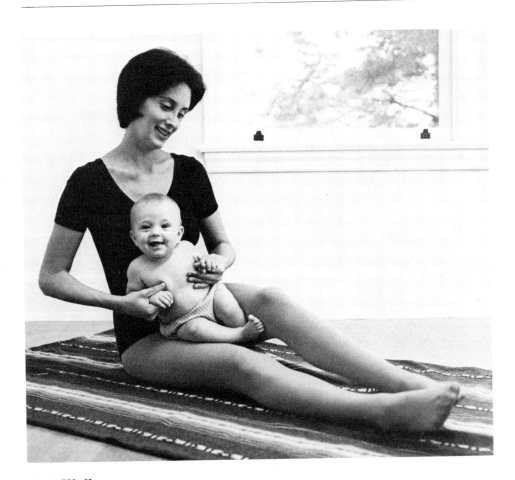

Butt Walker

Sit with your legs together and stretched forward. Place the baby in your lap.

Walk forward on your buttocks.

Walk backward, walk sideways. Vary your rhythm and speed.

This "walk" slims down your buttocks and strengthens the muscles in your lower back. My daughter loved this exercise, and in fact she still does it with me at two years of age. A variation is to rock from side to side (similar to *No Hips M'Lady* in Chapter 2).

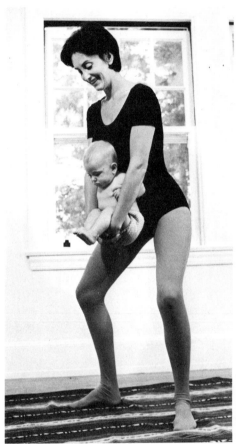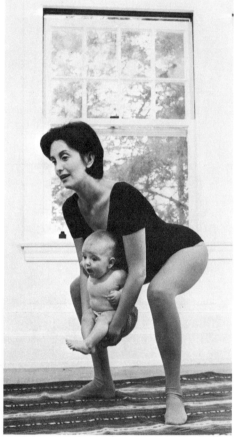

Squatting Swing

Hold the baby in your arms, hands clasped together. Exhale as you lower slowly down into a squat. Once your are securely balanced, swing your baby forward and back, lifting and lowering your buttocks. Breathe easily as you swing.

Slowly straighten your knees, holding the baby against your chest. Exhale, and continue to straighten your knees until you are standing tall.

Repeat the cycle of bending, swinging the baby, and straightening your knees.

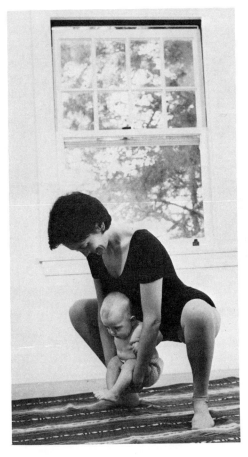

This is very similar to the squatting exercise you learned while pregnant. This exercise opens, strengthens, and stretches your inner thighs and helps to tone your perineum. With the added weight of the baby, you also stretch and strengthen your arms and legs. This is another exercise that is better started while your baby is still light. Babies love the ride.

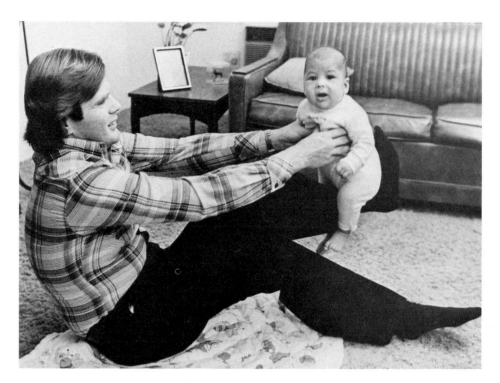

Ride 'Em Cowperson

Sit with knees bent, both feet flat on the floor.

Cross one leg over the other and sit the baby on your raised foot. Kick your leg, bouncing the baby gently.

Repeat with the other leg.

This exercise strengthens the muscles in your back, abdomen, knees, and lower leg.

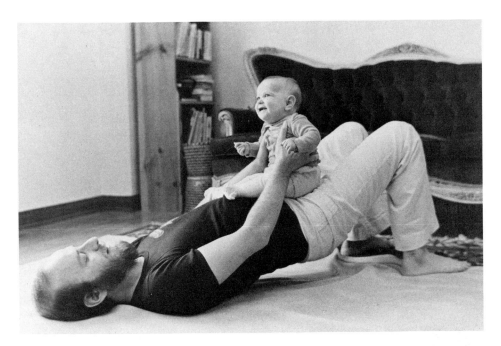

Pelvic Elevator

Lie on your back, knees bent, slightly apart, feet flat on the floor. Sit the baby on your lower abdomen. Exhale and slowly lift your buttocks off the floor, pressing down with your feet. Inhale and lower your buttocks to the floor. Repeat, raising your buttocks slightly higher each time. Holding your baby firmly, bounce your pelvis on the floor. Give your baby a ride!

This exercise tones the muscles in your upper thighs and abdomen.

New mothers need to go easy on the bouncy part. *Wait for at least two months after the birth before you begin this movement.* If the movement is too rough, the baby will react immediately. So watch for the baby's response.

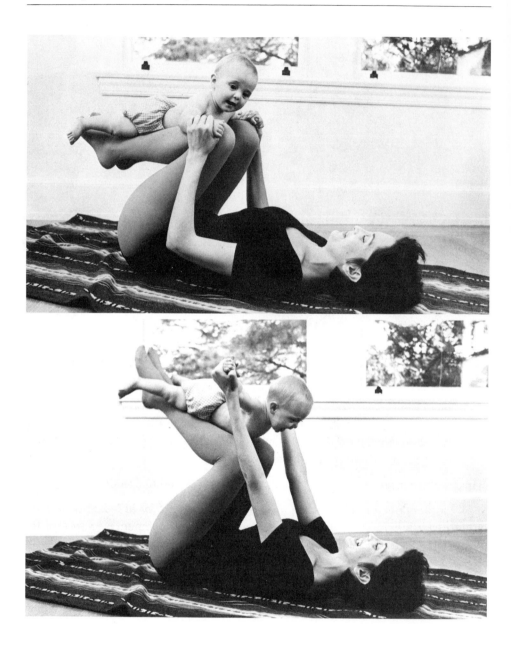

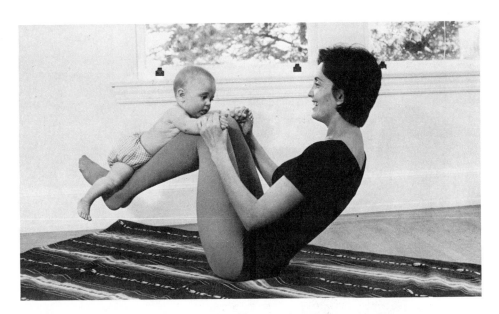

Rocking Horsey

Lie on your back, feet flat on the floor, legs together. Place the baby against your calves. Hold tight to her shoulders (for older babies, hold the hands).

Slowly lift your feet off the ground and extend the lower part of your legs. Stop when your calves are parallel with the floor. Exhale and pull your knees toward your chest. Inhale and push away. Continue to move your legs forward and back, moving the baby with a gentle rhythm.

Next, exhale and push your heels forward and "rock" up to a seated position. Place your feet flat on the floor, with knees still bent. Your baby will be standing up. Rock back gently, like a rocking horse, back and forth.

The first part of this exercise strengthens the muscles in your thighs and knees. The second part focuses on strengthening muscles in your lower back and abdomen. The third section relaxes your spine and strengthens the muscles in your abdomen and thighs.

Babies love this exercise. They get a chance to rock, stand up, and be lifted in the air. I loved watching Anna's expressions whenever we did this exercise. Somedays I wished I had a camera to catch the joy in her face.

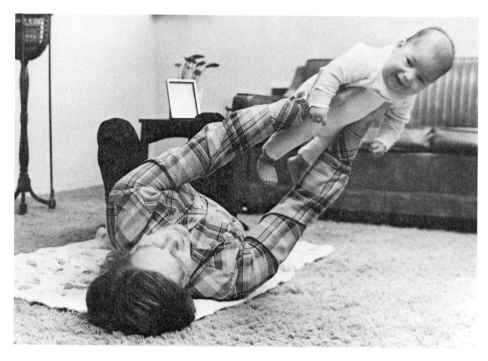

Barbell Baby

Lie on your back, knees bent, feet flat on the floor. Hold your baby firmly and try the variations listed below.

1. Exhale and lift the baby up off your chest. Inhale and lower the baby slowly.

2. Exhale, lift the baby, and move your arms all the way to the right. Rest your right upper arm on the floor. Inhale. Exhale, lift up and return to center. Repeat on the other side.

3. Exhale and raise the baby over your head. Inhale and bring her back to a resting position.

4. Make circles with your baby in the air. Begin with small circles, then let them get gradually larger. Reverse directions. Be aware of your breathing throughout the exercise.

This exercise is a prime example of how you can use the weight of your baby to tone your arms and back muscles. Each variation uses different muscles in your arms, shoulders, upper back, and chest. Experiment with variations of your own.

The earlier you start this exercise, the more likely you are to continue doing it as your baby grows heavier. To the baby, it feels like flying. Be aware of how fast you are moving. Think of baby's comfort too.

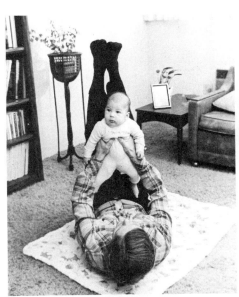 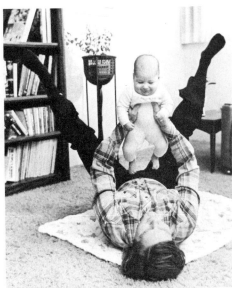

Scissors

Lie on your back with your legs off the ground. Hold the baby on your lower abdomen. (The baby can sit or stand, depending on his strength and age.) Exhale and bring your legs tight together.

Inhale and open your legs. As you open them, lift the baby in the air (make a sound). Exhale and cross one leg over the other, lowering the baby as you bring your legs together.

Repeat, crossing the opposite leg on top.

This exercise helps the muscles in both your arms and legs. The scissors action develops your inner and outer thigh muscles. Lifting your baby also builds your arm muscles. Babies love this one. They see you getting smaller and they feel bigger.

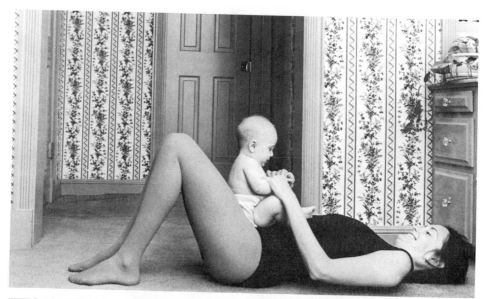

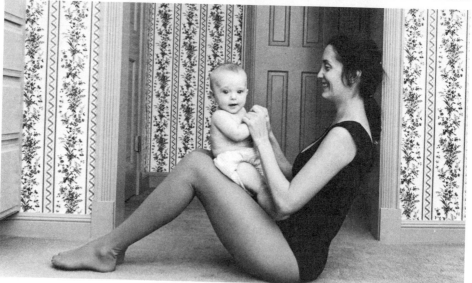

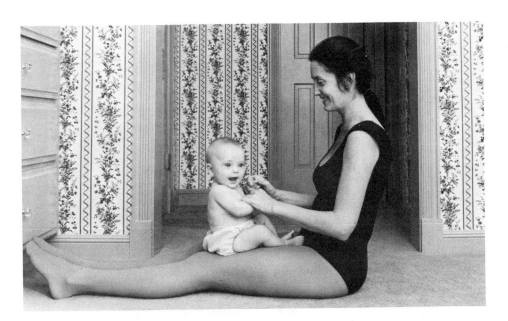

Sit-Ups

Lie on your back and place the baby on your lower abdomen. Bend your knees and place your feet flat on the floor.

Leave your knees bent and sit up, moving the baby onto your thighs. Slide your knees down and feel your spine lengthen.

Reverse the process to sit down: Slide your knees up, then slowly lower your back, one vertebra at a time, until your back is on the floor.

New mothers need to wait at least six weeks before doing this one. You do want your body to go back into place, especially your intestines and uterus, before you begin to strengthen your abdominals with a weight on top of them.

I loved to watch Anna's reaction to this exercise. It was as if she were saying, "Hey, how did we get up here?"

When you do this exercise, feel free to move your feet in any direction to help you sit up without strain. You will not only build your abdominal muscles, but can also strengthen your back muscles when you lower down slowly.

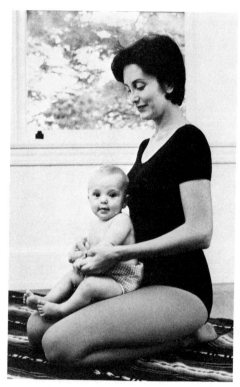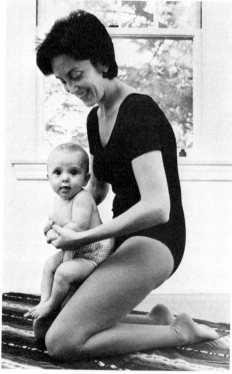

Thighs Guys

Sit with your legs folded underneath you, and place the baby in your lap. Tuck your pelvis under and feel as if a forklift is helping you lift your buttocks off your heels, just a little bit, as you exhale. Inhale and gently lower your buttocks back onto your heels.

This exercise is wonderful for strengthening your upper thighs—as well as your lower back and stomach if you include them in the lifting and lowering. For the baby it is definitely a ride, up and down on thighs that are getting stronger each time you do this exercise.

For many of us this exercise also helps the muscles feeding into the buttocks, which can and often do get flabby with lack of use. This exercise is great as an all-around toner for the pelvis. This is a must for getting back into shape.

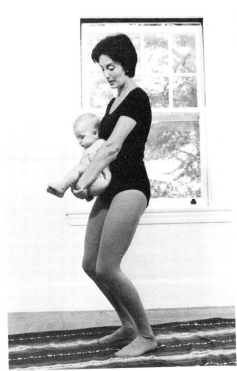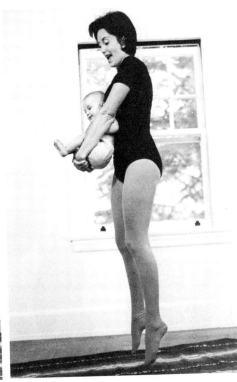

Up We Go

Hold the baby close to your body (as shown in the illustration, or in any other comfortable variation). Stand with your feet parallel, hip-width apart. Bend your knees slightly and jump lightly in the air. Repeat the jumps as high or as low as you have the strength to do.

Not only does this give the baby a chance to see the floor from quite a distance, but he gets a fun ride, while the parent strengthens the ankles and leg muscles and builds endurance in the knee joints.

The age of the baby will determine how high he likes to jump. As they get older, babies like it as high as you can go. What I love to do is have a line of parents jump toward each other and then jump away. When the babies are facing out, as in the photograph, they get to see what is happening. The joy on their faces makes this exercise a treat for everyone.

243

Epilogue

Ending the book presents its own challenge. With every class I teach, a new exercise gets created and I want to add it to the book, but I have to stop somewhere. You have just finished the process of pregnancy and birth and are now embarking on the journey of parenting. There are a wealth of resources in your own community for you to explore. Look for local classes for new parents, infant gym classes, or exercise classes for new mothers. There is more and more being offered each year. Contact your church or local YWCA or YMCA; they are often rich sources of classes or information about support groups. If you happen to live in a place where not much is happening, create your own group. You can use this book as a starting tool. Let your imagination and playfulness create your own program, tailored to your specific group. Picnics and other outdoor activities can offer a place to gather and share, especially during the warm months. Find a living room that is large enough to create a class space. Your alternatives are all there. Allow yourself to explore them wherever you live.

At this special time in your life, I wish you and your family good health, and a wonderful time creating your own Baby Dance!

Resource guide

The organizations listed here are support groups which offer information, classes, literature, and in some cases training programs to certify childbirth educators.

American Academy of Husband-Coached Childbirth (Bradley information)
Post Office Box 5224
Sherman Oaks, California 91413

American Public Health Association
Section on Maternal and Child Health
1790 Broadway
New York, New York 10023

American Society for Psychoprophylaxis in Obstetrics (Lamaze information)
1523 L Street, N.W. or 1411 K Street, N.W.
Washington, D.C. 20005
(202) 783-7050

Baby Dance Productions
Elysa Markowitz
4061 Wade Street, Apt. A
Los Angeles, California 90066
         Exercise posters & tapes, films, and Anna's birth slides are available.

Holistic Childbirth Institute
1627 Tenth Avenue
San Francisco, California 94122
(415) 664-1119

International Childbirth Education Association, Inc.
Post Office Box 20852
Milwaukee, Wisconsin 53220
Supplies Center: Post Office Box 70258, Seattle, Washington 98107

La Leche League International
9616 Minneapolis Avenue
Franklin Park, Illinois 60131

Maternity Center Association
48 East 92nd Street
New York, New York 10028

Society for the Protection of the Unborn through Nutrition (SPUN)
Suite 603
17 N. Wabash
Chicago, Illinois 60602

HOME BIRTH RESOURCES

Association for Childbirth at Home International (ACHI)
Post Office Box 1219
Cerritos, California 90701

Homebirth, Inc.
89 Franklin Street
Suite 200
Boston, Massachusetts 92110
(617) 482-8175

Informed Homebirth
Box 788
Boulder, Colorado 80306
(303) 444-0434

National Association for Parents and Professionals for Safe Alternatives in
Childbirth (NAPSAC)
P. O. Box 267
Marble Hill, Missouri 63764

CESAREAN BIRTH RESOURCES

CARESS: Cesarean Association for Research, Education, Support and
        Satisfaction in Birthing
11919 Ashdale Lane
Studio City, California 91604
(213) 674-5227

C-Birth Association
125 North 12th Street
New Hyde Park, New York 11040

C/Birth: The Cesarean Birth Association of Southern California
2407 North Louise Street
Santa Ana, California 92706

C/Sec
15 Maynard Road
Dedham, Massachusetts 02026

Cesarean Support Group of New York
184 Elm Avenue
Teaneck, New Jersey 07666

Bibliography

The following is a list of books I have found helpful in my journey of learning about pregnancy and parenting. If you are unable to find any of the books listed below, please refer to the Resource Guide on page 245–247.

PREGNANCY AND BIRTH

Arms, Suzanne, *Immaculate Deception*. New York: Bantam Books, 1975.

Bing, Elizabeth, and Libby Colman, *Making Love During Pregnancy*. New York: Bantam, 1977.

Bradley, Robert, M.D., *Husband-Coached Childbirth*. New York: Harper & Row, 1974.

Brook, Danae, *Naturebirth: You, Your Body, and Your Baby*. New York: Pantheon Books, 1976.

Colman, Arthur, and Libby Colman, *Pregnancy: The Psychological Experience*. New York: Bantam Books, 1971.

Dick-Read, Grantly, *Childbirth Without Fear*. New York: Harper & Row, 1959.

Ewy, Donna, and Roger Ewy, *Preparation for Childbirth*. Boulder, Colo.: Pruett, 1970.

Hazell, Lester Dessez, *Commonsense Childbirth*. New York: Berkeley, 1976.

Kitzinger, Sheila, *The Experience of Childbirth*, 4th ed. New York: Penguin, 1978.

——, *Giving Birth: The Parents' Emotions in Childbirth*. New York: Schocken, 1977.

LeBoyer, Frederick, M.D., *Birth Without Violence*. New York: Knopf, 1975.

Milinaire, Catherine, *Birth*. New York: Crown, 1974.

Simpkins, Penny, and Margot Edwards, "When Your Baby Has Jaundice" (pamphlet), Penny Press, Seattle, 1979.

HOME BIRTH

Baldwin, Rahima, *Special Delivery*. Millbrae, Calif.: Les Femmes Publishing, 1979.

Brooks, Tonya, and Linda Bennett, *Giving Birth at Home*. Cerritos, Calif.: Association for Childbirth at Home, International, 1977.

Gaskin, Ina May, *Spiritual Midwifery*. Summertown, Tenn.: The Book Publishing Company, 1978.

Gold, E. J., and Cybele Gold, *Joyous Childbirth: Manual for Conscious Natural Childbirth*. Berkeley, Calif.: And/Or Press, 1977.

Hathaway, Marjie, and Jay Hathaway, *Children at Birth*. Sherman Oaks, Calif.: Academy Publications, 1978.

Lang, Raven, *Birth Book*. Palo Alto, Calif. Genesis Press, 1972.

Smoke, Stephen, ed., *Dr. Ettinghausen's Skilled Childbirth at Home*. Van Nuys, Calif.: Smoke & Bruce Publishing, 1975.

Sousa, Marion, *Childbirth at Home*. Englewood Cliffs, N.J.: Prentice-Hall, 1976.

Stewart, David, and Lee Stewart, eds., *Safe Alternatives in Childbirth*. Chapel Hill, N.C.: NAPSAC, 1977.

Ward, Charlotte, and Fred Ward, *The Home Birth Book*, New York: Doubleday, 1977.

White, Gregory, M.D., *Emergency Childbirth*. Franklin Park, Ill.: Police Training Foundation, 1958.

FETAL GROWTH AND DEVELOPMENT

Caveney, Sylvia, *Inside Mom*. New York: St. Martin's Press, 1976.

Nilsson, Lenart, Axel Ingelman-Sundberg, and Claes Wirsen, *A Child Is Born*. New York: Delacorte Press, 1978.

Rugh, Roberts, and Landrum B. Shettles, M.D., *From Conception to Birth*. New York: Harper & Row, 1971.

EXERCISE BOOKS

Mom

Dilfer, Carol, *Your Baby, Your Body*. New York: Crown, 1977.

Hartman, Rhondda, *Exercises for True Natural Childbirth*. New York: Harper & Row, 1975.

LeBoyer, Frederick, M.D., *Inner Beauty, Inner Light*, New York: Knopf, 1978.

Medvin, Jeannine, *Prenatal Yoga and Natural Birth*. Berkeley, Calif.: Freestone, 1974.

Nobel, Elizabeth, *Essential Exercises for the Childbearing Years*. Boston: Houghton Mifflin, 1976.

Thompson, Judi, *Healthy Pregnancy: The Yoga Way*. New York: Dolphin, 1977.

Baby

Levy, Janine, M.D., *The Baby Exercise Book*. New York: Pantheon, 1973.

Prudden, Bonnie, *How to Keep Your Child Fit from Birth to Six*. New York: Harper & Row, 1964.

Timmermans, Claire, *How to Teach Your Baby to Swim*. New York: Stein and Day, 1976.

Cesarean Birth

Heilman, Joan Rattner, *Having a Cesarean Baby*. New York: Dutton, 1978.

FOR EXPECTANT FATHERS

Bittman, Sam, and Sue Rosenberg Zalk, Ph.D., *Expectant Fathers*. New York: Hawthorn Books, 1978.

NUTRITION

Brewer, Gail, and Tom Brewer, M.D., *What Every Pregnant Woman Should Know*, New York, Penguin, 1977.
Davis, Adelle, *Let's Have Healthy Children*. New York: Signet, 1972.
Dotzler, Louise, ed., *The Farm Vegetarian Cookbook*. Summertown, Tenn.: The Book Publishing Company, 1978.
Ewald, Ellen, *Recipes for a Small Planet*. New York: Ballantine, 1973.
Kirschmann, John D., *Nutrition Almanac*. New York: McGraw-Hill, 1975.
Lappe, Frances, *Diet for a Small Planet*. New York: Ballantine, 1971.
Shurtleff, William, and Akiko Aoyagi, *The Book of Tofu*. Brookline, Mass.: Autumn Press, 1975.

BREASTFEEDING

Carson, Mary B., ed., *Womanly Art of Breastfeeding*. Franklin Park, Ill.: La Leche League International, 1963.
Kippley, Sheila, *Breast-feeding and Natural Child Spacing*. New York: Harper & Row, 1974.
Pryor, Karen, *Nursing Your Baby*. rev. ed. New York: Pocket Books, 1973.

HERBS

Grieve, M., *A Modern Herbal,* 2 vols. New York: Dover Publications, 1971.
Parvati, Jeanine, *Hygieia: A Woman's Herbal*. Berkeley, Calif.: Book People, 1978.

CHILDREN AND PARENTS

Berends, Polly, *Whole Child, Whole Parent*. New York: Harper Magazine Press, 1975.

Boston Women's Health Book Collective, *Ourselves and Our Children*. New York: Random House, 1978.

Brazelton, T. Berry, M.D., *Infants and Mothers: Differences in Development*. New York: Dell, 1976.

———, *Toddlers and Parents*. New York, Dell, 1976.

Gordon, Thomas, *P.E.T. Parent Effectiveness Training*. New York: Plume Books, 1975.

Green, Martin I., *A Sigh of Relief: The First-Aid Handbook for Childhood Emergencies*. New York: Bantam, 1977.

LeBoyer, Frederick, M.D., *Loving Hands*. New York: Knopf, 1976.

Meyers, Carole, *How to Organize a Babysitting Cooperative and Get Some Free Time Away from the Kids*. Albany, Calif.: Carousel, 1976.

Montagu, Ashley, *Touching: The Significance of the Skin*. New York: Columbia University Press, 1971.

Pearce, Joseph Chilton, *Magical Child*. New York: E. P. Dutton, 1977.

Thevenin, Tine, *The Family Bed: An Age-Old Concept in Child Rearing*. Minneapolis: Thevenin, 1976.

WOMEN'S HEALTH

Boston Women's Health Book Collective, *Our Bodies, Ourselves*. New York: Simon & Schuster, 1973.

Carter, Mildred, *Hand Reflexology: The Key to Perfect Health*. Los Angeles: Parker, 1975.

Deutsch, Ronald, *The Key to Feminine Response in Marriage*. New York: Ballantine, 1968.

Nofziger, Margaret, *A Cooperative Method of Natural Birth Control*. Summertown, Tenn.: The Book Publishing Company, 1976.